The Miracle of
NUTS, SEEDS AND GRAINS

The Miracle of
NUTS, SEEDS AND GRAINS

The Scientific Facts about Nutritional
Properties and Medicinal Values of
Nuts, Seeds and Grains

Dr Bahram Tadayyon,
MNS, MD, Ph.D.

Library of Congress Control Number:		2013911878
ISBN:	Hardcover	978-1-4836-6175-9
	Softcover	978-1-4836-6174-2
	Ebook	978-1-4836-6176-6

The contents of this book are to be used for educational purposes only and should not be regarded as a substitute for the medical advice of your own doctor.

The author is not liable for any treatment performed by a user based on the contents of this book.

Rev. date: 06/28/2013

To order additional copies of this book, contact:
Xlibris Corporation
1-800-455-039
www.Xlibris.com.au
Orders@Xlibris.com.au
504147

CONTENTS

DEDICATION

I dedicate this book to my better half, *Heba,* whose constant encouragement, support, and patience made writing this manuscript possible.

A handful of nuts a day will keep doctors away.
So go 'nuts' and become 'nutty'.

(Dr Bahram Tadayyon)

INTRODUCTION

You agree with me that health is the greatest wealth; otherwise, you would not have picked up this book to read.

As is evident from my two previous books, *The Miracle of Fruits* and *The Miracle of Vegetables*, my goal in writing these series of books is to increase public awareness about the health benefits of natural foods.

Nuts, seeds, and grains not only add pleasure and variety to our diets but also prevent numerous chronic diseases and cure many ailments naturally, avoiding drug side effects.

NUTS

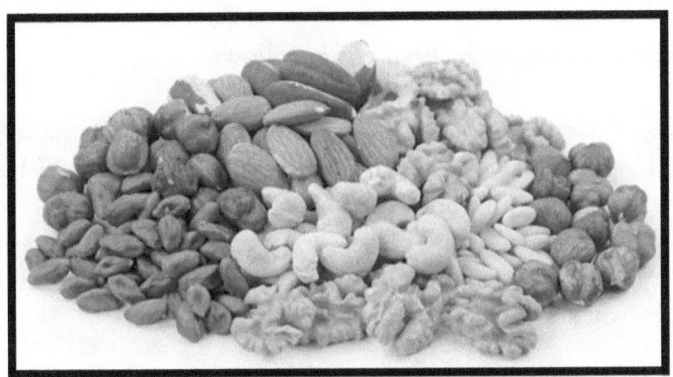

Nuts are delicious gifts to mankind from Mother Nature.

A nut is the dry one-seeded fruit of trees or shrubs, consisting of an edible kernel in a hard shell that protects the embryo from the surrounding environment.

A nut is a specific type of seed that has a hard external wall and does not open to release its seed at maturity.

Common usage of the term nut refers to any hard-walled edible kernel.

Nuts are oily and crunchy. They have been an important part of human diet for thousands of years.

Classification of Nuts
Nuts can be classified according to the following families:

Beech family: Chestnut, chinquapin
Birch family: Hazelnut
Cashew family: Cashew, pistachio
Legume family: Peanuts

Pine family: Pine
Protea family: Macadamia
Sapucaia family: Brazil nut, paradise nut
Walnut family: Hickory nut, pecan, walnut

Serving Size of Nuts
A serving size of nuts is 1 oz, which is about a handful.

The number of nuts in each serving is as follows:

24 almonds, 4 Brazil nuts, 15 cashews, 28 peanuts, 8 macadamias, 45 pistachios, 15 pecan halves, 15 walnut halves, 6 chestnuts, 25 hazelnuts, 3 tablespoons pine nuts, and one-third of a cup soy nuts. It is recommended to eat 1.5 oz of nuts per day. However, if you are watching your weight, you must try not to exceed 50 g per day, although it is difficult to control yourself once you start eating the delicious nuts.

Nuts can be eaten as snacks, salad toppings, desserts, confectionaries, and as flavouring and garnishing for various dishes. Nut oils are used in cooking, cosmetics, and pharmaceuticals.

Fresh versus Roasted Nuts

Eating fresh raw nuts is preferable over oil-roasted or honey-covered nuts, which add calories, or salted nuts, which add sodium. Roasted nuts might have been heated in unhealthy hydrogenated fats or at high temperature that can destroy their nutrients.

Health Benefits of Nuts

Nuts are small in size but are powerhouses of nutrients. Although this varies from nut to nut, most nuts contain at least some of the following benefits:

1. Nut eaters have higher good cholesterol, lower bad cholesterol, and lower C-reactive protein, a marker of inflammation in the body. Nuts are one of the best plant-based sources of Omega-3 fatty acids that prevent dangerous heart rhythm that could lead to heart attack. Vitamin E in nuts stops development of plaques in arteries,

which narrows them. Some nuts contain plant sterols that lower cholesterol. Arginine in some nuts improves the health of artery walls by making them more flexible and less prone to blood clots that can block blood flow. All nuts contain a high amount of fibre that lower cholesterol.

2. Fibre and fats in nuts create a sense of fullness, suppressing appetite, thus leading to weight loss.
3. Vitamin E and Omega fatty acids in nuts improve hair and nail quality.
4. Nuts protect against certain cancers.
5. Nuts boost overall longevity.
6. Nuts are rich in high-quality proteins, antioxidants, some minerals, and B vitamins.
7. Nuts have a low glycaemic index, making them useful for diabetics.
8. Nuts have high energy content and contain a lot of fat (as much as 80 per cent), most of which is healthy but is high in calories. Hence, nuts should be consumed in moderation.

Nut Oil

Nut oils are good sources of Omega-3 fatty acids and vitamin E but lack fibre. Nut oils contain saturated as well as unsaturated fatty acids. They are good to use in salad dressing and cooking, but if overcooked, they can become bitter. They should be used in moderation because they are high in calories. Nut oils are also used in massage treatment, aromatherapy, cosmetics, and pharmaceuticals.

When Not To Become 'Nutty'?

One to two percentage of the world's population are allergic to nuts. Wait until children are at least one-year-old before introducing them to any kind of nut.

ALPHABETICAL LIST OF NUTS

Acorn
Almond
Barking deer's mango nut
Bat nut
Beechnut
Betel nut
Brazil nut
Breadnut
Candlenut
Cashew
Chestnut
Chinquapin
Coco de mer
Coconut
Ginkgo nut
Hazelnut

Kluwak nut
Kola nut
Macadamia
Mamoncillo
Mongongo
Ogbono
Paradise nut
Peanut
Pecan
Pekea nut
Pili nut
Pine nut
Pistachio
Soy nut
Tiger nut
Walnut

ACORN (OAK NUT)

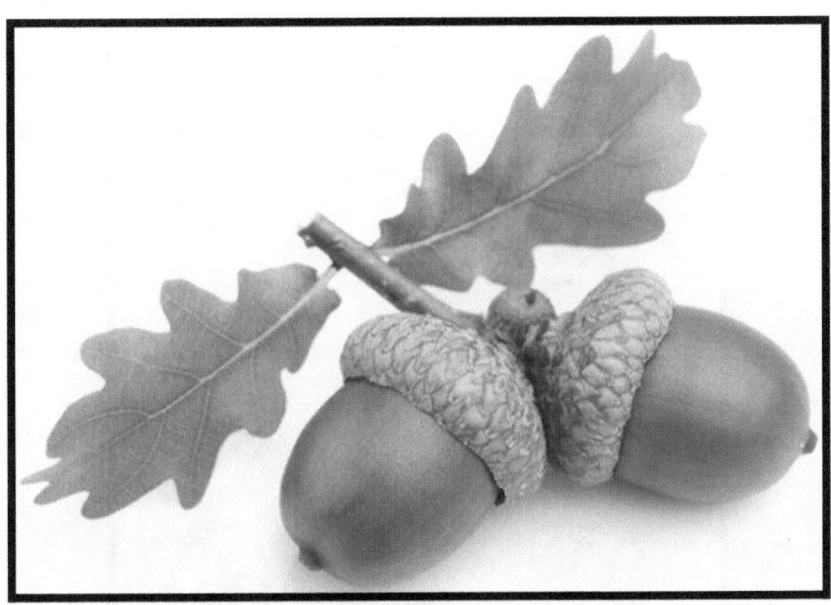

Acorn is the nut of oaks. A long time ago, it was a staple diet of Native Americans and Koreans and served as a food source for many cultures around the world. Most people rarely eat it because they associate it with the food of squirrels.

Acorn is the symbol for the National Trails of England and Wales.

Acorn usually contains a simple seed, enclosed in a tough leathery shell. Because of its high tannin content, it requires some preparation to make it palatable.

Acorn is not as high in fats as other nuts. It contains fibre, complex carbohydrates, B vitamins, manganese, copper, and magnesium.

Acorn can be processed into flour to make baked goods such as breads, muffins, cookies, soups, toppings for desserts, and as a coffee substitute.

One of the benefits of eating acorn is its association with controlling blood sugar level.

ALMONDS

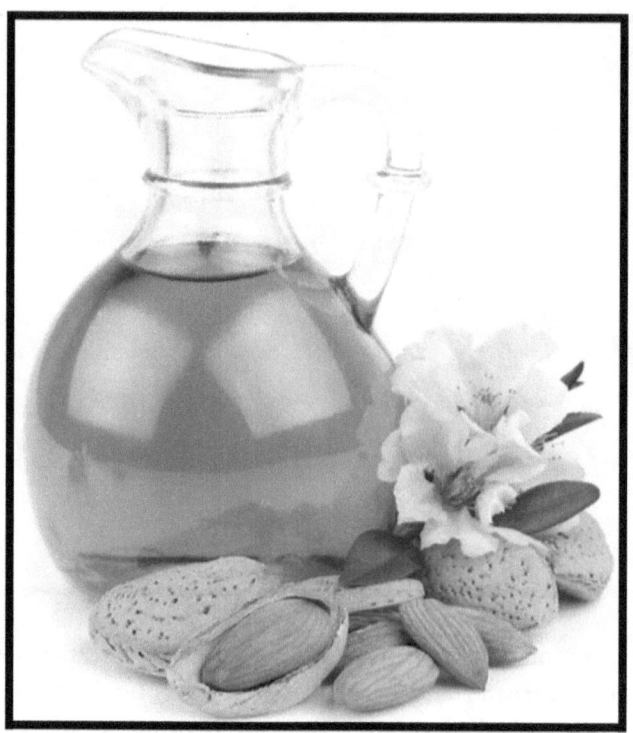

Almond is the seed of the fruit of the almond tree related to peach, cherry, and plum. Almonds originated in Western Asia and North Africa. The largest producer of almonds today is the United States. Almonds are one of the oldest nuts and have been written about in many historical texts, including the Bible. They are off-white in colour, covered by a thin brownish skin protected by a hard shell. Sweet almond is oval with a crunchy texture and buttery flavour. Bitter almond is used to make oil, which is used as a flavouring agent for foods and liqueurs and in lotions.

Almond can be eaten raw, as almond milk, rice dishes, curries, desserts, confectionaries, and almond butter. Green almonds are eaten as snacks in Iran.

Almond skin contains more than 20 antioxidant flavonoids. One ounce (23 nuts) contains 163 calories, 14 g fats, and 4 g fibre. It is a rich source of protein, tryptophan, monounsaturated fatty acids, vitamin E (more than any other nut), riboflavin, copper, manganese, magnesium, potassium, calcium, phosphorus, iron, and selenium.

Some of the benefits of eating almonds are that they

1. have high content of copper, manganese, and riboflavin that help in energy production.
2. have monounsaturated fatty acids that satisfy appetite and prevent overeating.
3. have the antioxidants vitamin E and selenium that eliminate toxins and free radicals from the body.
4. have fibre that prevents constipation, haemorrhoids, and colon cancer and also blocks absorption of some of the fats present in the nut.
5. contain vitamin E that nourishes skin and helps improve complexion.
6. decrease rise in glucose and insulin levels, and thus help people suffering from type 2 diabetes.
7. have high potassium and low sodium contents that help in lowering blood pressure.
8. contain high monounsaturated fatty acids (70 per cent of the almond fat) that help maintain a healthy heart by lowering bad cholesterol and increasing good cholesterol. Vitamin E and flavonoids help prevent heart diseases.
9. contain calcium, phosphorus, and magnesium that help build strong bones and teeth.
10. have riboflavin and l-carnitine that boost brain activity and lower the risk of Alzheimer's disease.
11. are the only nut that is alkaline-forming; thus, it prevents osteoporosis, poor immunity, low energy, and weight gain.

Almond Oil

Almond oil is used as an emollient, as a skin and hair moisturiser, in cooking, as a carrier or base in aromatherapy, and in cosmetic and pharmaceutical industries. It is also great for body massage. It lowers the appearance of acne, blackheads, and whiteheads. Almond oil is good for cooking at high temperatures as it has a high smoking point.

Bat Nut

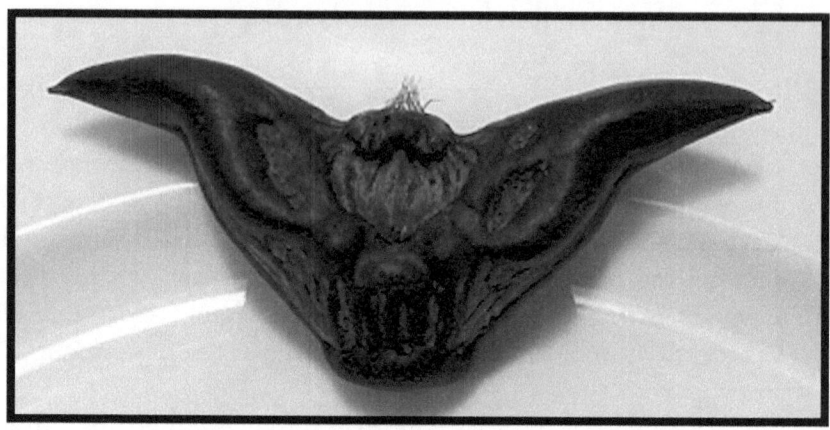

Bat nut is also known as water caltrop, water chestnut, goat head, buffalo nut, and devil pod.

It is a floating aquatic Asian plant that resembles the head of a bull. It contains a single large starchy seed. The shell is very tough and brittle. It has a putrid smell and could be infested with worms.

Bat nut could be eaten boiled, roasted, or powdered and added to other foods. It tastes like chestnut. The texture of the cooked nut is powdery and starchy.

Bat nut appears on my list of the world's five most unusual nuts.

Barking Deer's Mango Nut

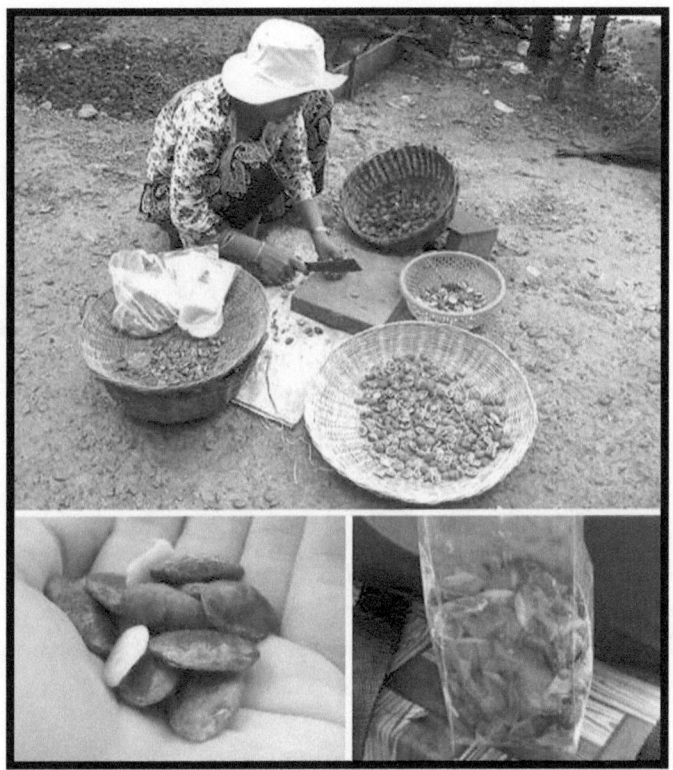

It is also known as cha bok and cow's favourite; it is actually not a nut but a seed from the pit of a sour fruit eaten in Southeast Asia. It gets its strange name from observation that it is the favourite food of the barking deer, native to Southeast Asia.

It is also called cow's favourite because it passes intact through the digestive tract of cows.

The bitter astringent shell is peeled off before eating. Underneath the thin brown skin, a delicious, smooth, buttery white aromatic flesh appears that tastes like a cross between peanuts and macadamia nuts.

It appears on my list of the world's most unusual nuts.

BEECHNUTS

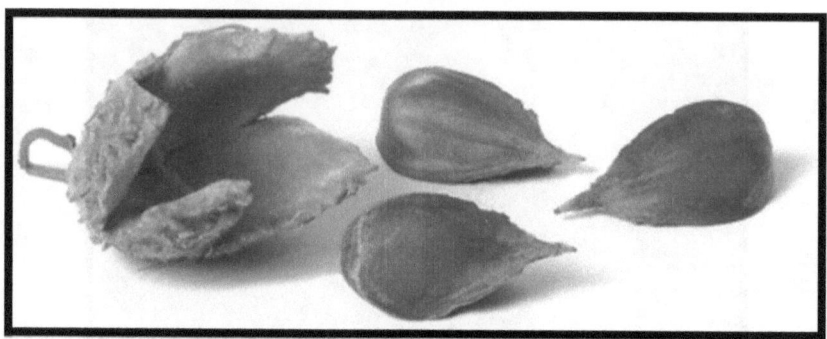

Beechnuts are native to temperate Eurasia and North America. Following pollination, beech tree produces triangle-shaped fruits that hang midair in groups of two to three. The edible fruit is referred to as beechnut and has sweet white kernel.

Beechnuts are one of the most delicious of all wild nuts but are not as widely used by humans as other nuts because they are difficult to remove from the shells and have high tannin content. However, they support a wide variety of wildlife, including deer, squirrels, raccoons, and pigs.

Beechnuts have 22 per cent protein and can be ground to powder and made into bread or can be roasted and used as a substitute for coffee.

Betel Nut

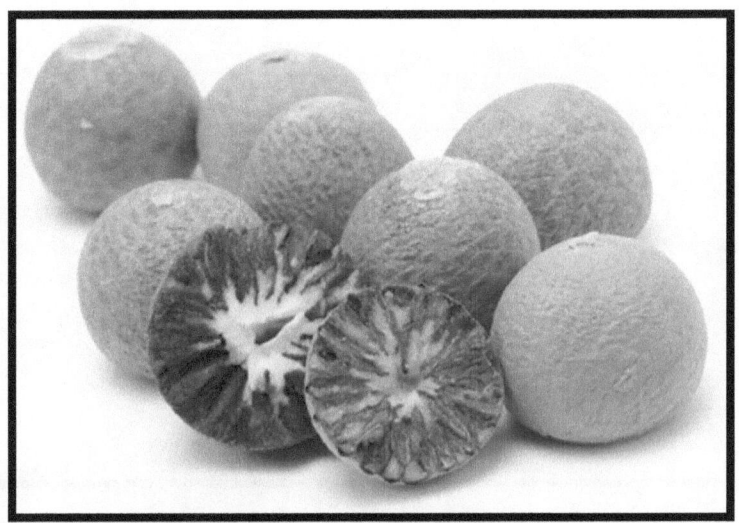

Areca nut is the seed of the areca palm, which grows in the Pacific, Asia, and East Africa. It is referred to as betel nut because it is often chewed wrapped in betel leaves (which have peppery bitter taste) along with powdered lime, flavouring agents (like clove, cardamom, and catchin), and occasionally tobacco. This combination is called 'paan' in Asia. It is chewed for its psychoactive and stimulant effects by about 5 per cent of the world's population, which is more than the use of chewing gums. Its eight closely related alkaloids are responsible for the stimulant effect. It is popular in ceremonies for its effect in causing warmth and heightened alertness.

It stimulates intestinal peristalsis, aids in digestion, relieves dry mouth, prevents dental cavity by its antibacterial effect, and improves symptoms of schizophrenia.

However, in Western cultures, it is not accepted because the chewers spit out the red saliva.

Its drawbacks include increasing the risk of certain cancers (oral cavity, oesophagus, and stomach) and worsening the symptoms of blood pressure, irregular heartbeat, and asthma.

Brazil Nuts

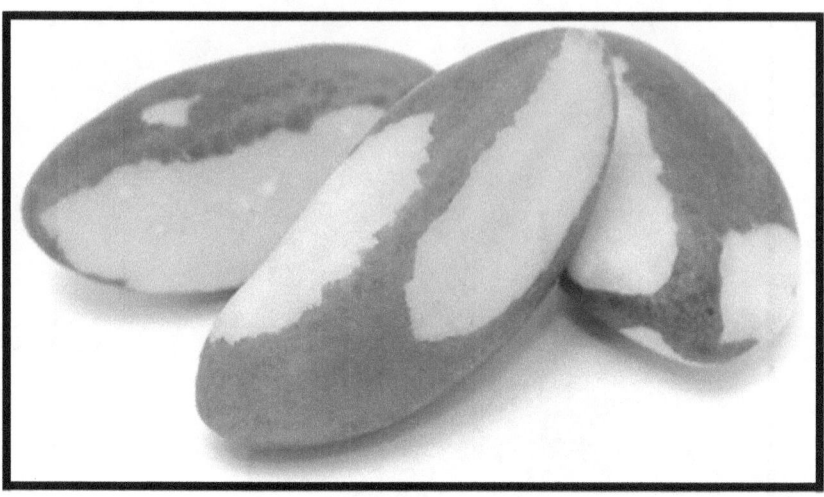

Brazil nut is botanically not a nut but a seed from the fruit of the tree. Despite its name, the greatest exporter of Brazil nut is not Brazil but Bolivia. Brazil nuts are native to South America. The trees grow up to 165 feet in height in the Amazon forests and produce tons of sweet yellowish flowers and fruits. Brazil nut has a woody thick shell, inside of which are buttery nuts with brown skin. Its texture is smooth, and its taste is sweet, similar to macadamia nut.

Like other nuts, Brazil nuts have high nutrient content. They contain 18 per cent protein, 13 per cent carbohydrates, 69 per cent fats, fibre, vitamins (D, C, and B), and minerals (selenium, phosphorus, magnesium, calcium, copper, iron, manganese, and zinc). One ounce of Brazil nut (6 kernels) has 186 calories, 2 g fibre, and 19 g fat. Compared to other nuts, Brazil nut has the highest concentration of saturated fats (25 per cent).

Some of the benefits of eating Brazil nuts are that they

1. are the best source of selenium. One single kernel provides 100 per cent of the daily requirement for this nutrient. Selenium promotes healthy immune system, improves thyroid gland function, lowers joint inflammation, and prevents certain cancers.

2. lower bad cholesterol and help prevent heart attack and stroke.
3. lower the risk of several cancers, including prostate, breast, stomach, colon, and lung cancer.
4. boost immunity and fight infection.
5. boost fertility.
6. provide all the essential amino acids needed for human growth and development.
7. have a high amino acid methionine that prevents liver cirrhosis, heart diseases, and premature ageing.
8. have a high fibre content that prevents constipation and colon cancer.

Disadvantagescontain a high concentration of phytic acid which prevents absorption of some nutrients, especially iron.

1. can be toxic in overdose, causing nail damage, hair fall, fatigue, rash, irritability, and stomach upset.
2. contain aflatoxin, which is carcinogenic.
3. contain a small amount of radioactive radium because of their vast root system.
4. produce allergies in some people.
5. become rancid fast because of their high content of polyunsaturated fats.

Breadnut (Maya Nut)

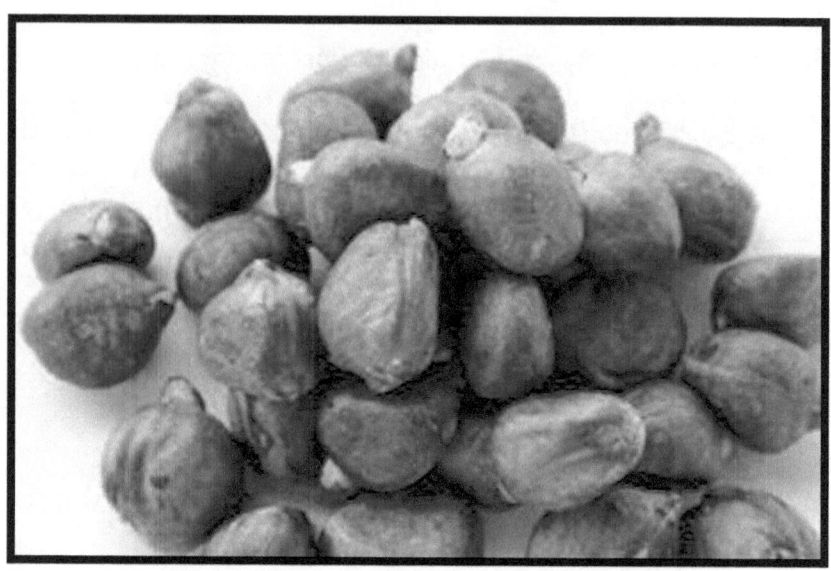

Breadnut is related to mulberries and figs. It is grown mainly in South America.

Breadnut has a large seed covered by a tasty citrus-flavoured orange-coloured skin that can be boiled or dried and ground to make porridge or bread. After boiling, it tastes like mashed potato, but after roasting, it tastes like coffee or chocolate.

Breadnut is a rich source of fibre, protein, vitamin B, antioxidants, calcium, potassium, iron, and zinc.

Breadnut has a low glycaemic index, making it suitable for people with type 2 diabetes.

CANDLENUT

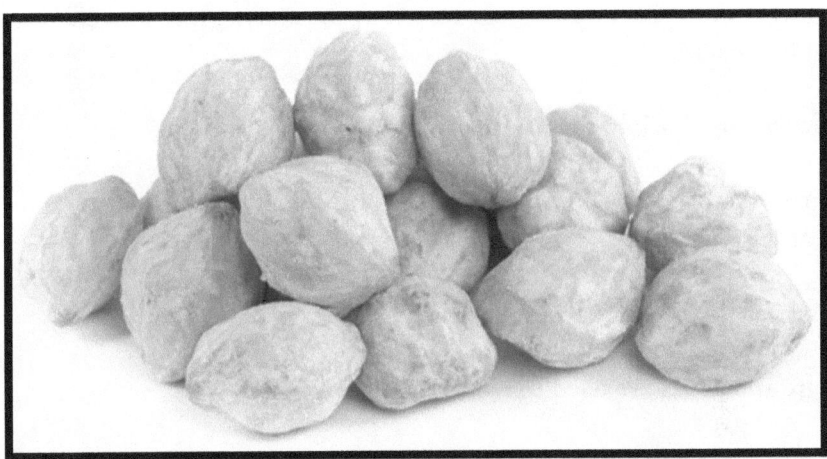

Candlenut is also known as Indian walnut, candleberry, and kukui nut. It gets its name from its ability to burn and give off light like a candle, which is the result of the highly inflammable oil content of the seed. In Hawaii, it is known as kukui, meaning lightning. Candlenut trees are indigenous to Southeast Asia and Hawaii and are cultivated in South America and Australia.

The tree can produce up to 180 pounds of nuts. The nuts are the size of chestnuts and have hard green or brown shells with a creamy pulp, containing one or two soft elliptical cream-coloured seeds.

The nuts have a bitter taste, and because of their saponin and phorbol content, they are mildly toxic if eaten raw.

Candlenut is used as an ingredient in Asian, Hawaiian, and South American cuisines.

Candlenut is a rich source of fibre, protein, healthy fats, vitamin B, minerals (potassium, phosphorus, magnesium, calcium, iron, zinc, copper, and selenium), saponins, flavonoids, and phytosterols. Every part of the candlenut tree has practical value. Because of its numerous roles in Hawaiian culture, candlenut has been designated the official state tree of Hawaii.

The oil is applied to the scalp to stimulate hair growth. It is used like castor oil to treat constipation. It is taken as a weight loss supplement and as a cholesterol-lowering agent. It is effective in relieving the pain from arthritis.

The leaves are used in poultices to relieve headache, fever, swollen joints, and skin ulcers.

The leaves and bark have antimicrobial properties.

In Japan, the bark is used to treat various tumours. In Java, the bark is used to treat dysentery.

The flower is used to treat oral thrush.

The ground seeds are used to treat skin ulcers.

In Hawaii, the trunk is used to make canoes, which are then varnished with candlenut oil.

The nuts are charred and made into an ink, which is used for tattoos.

Nuts are made into paste and used as soap or shampoo.

Candlenut appears on my list of five most unusual nuts.

CASHEWS

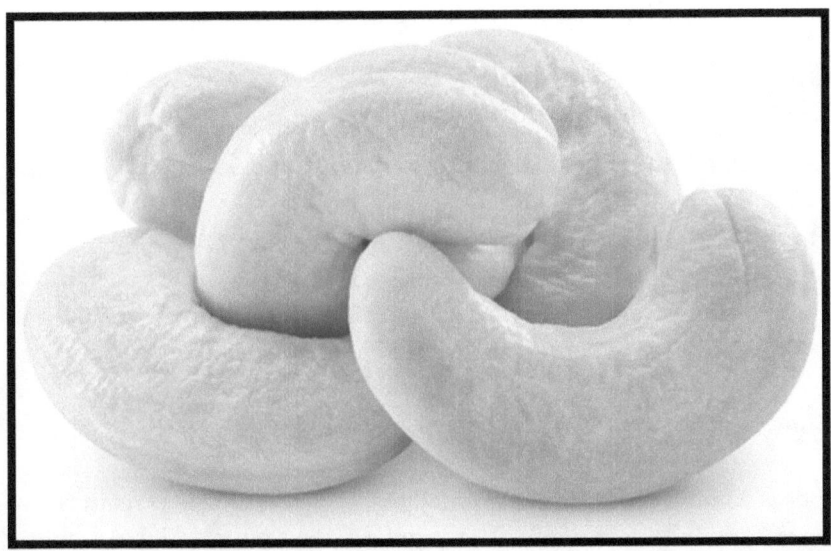

Cashew nut is a kidney or bean-shaped seed or fruit that grows on a tree about 30 feet tall in a double shell at the end of the cashew apple. Unlike other nuts, cashews are not sold inside their shells which contain a poisonous resin related to the poison ivy family, called cashew balm. This resin must be removed before the nut is consumed. Cashew is a close relative of pistachio and mango.

Cashews are native to Brazil, but today, the leading producers are India, Brazil, some African countries, and Vietnam.

Cashews have creamy-white buttery texture, smooth surface, sweet flavour, and fruity aroma. They are consumed raw or added to stir-fries, salads, and desserts.

One ounce of cashew (17 kernels) contains 180 calories, 14 g fat, 5 g protein, 8 g carbohydrates, 2 g fibre, minerals (magnesium, copper, phosphorus, manganese, zinc, selenium, and iron), tryptophan, phytosterols, and antioxidants. Its fat is unsaturated, mostly oleic acid, which promotes cardiovascular health.

Cancer Prevention

Proanthocyanidins in cashew nuts are flavonols that starve tumours and stop cancer cells from dividing. The fibre lowers colon cancer risk. High copper eliminates free radicals which could cause cancer.

Energy

Cashews are relatively high in energy, contributing 553 calories/100 g.

Heart Health

High oleic acid lowers the level of triglycerides. High antioxidants lower the risk of heart disease. Magnesium lowers blood pressure.

Hair and Skin Health

Copper is a component of many enzymes, one of which is tyrosinase, which converts tyrosine to melanin, the pigment that gives hair and skin their colour.

Eye Health

Cashews contain a small quantity of zeaxanthin, a flavonoid antioxidant pigment that protects eye from macular degeneration in the elderly.

Bone Health

Cashew is rich in several minerals that are involved in strong bone formation.

Nerve Health

Magnesium relaxes nerves and lowers the frequency of migraine attacks.

CHESTNUTS

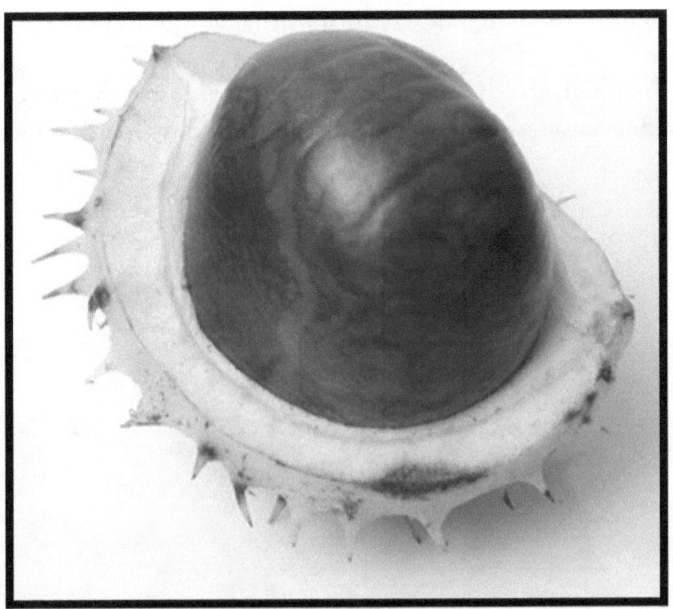

Chestnuts are native to hilly forests of China, Japan, Korea, Mediterranean region, Europe, and North America. Native Americans used it for centuries as a staple food like potato.

Chestnuts have smooth, glossy dark-brown shell with two to three orange-white, sweet, and starchy kernels. Unlike other tree nuts, the inside of chestnuts is not hard, but soft and fleshy, and cannot be eaten raw because it contains very high amount of tannic acids, which can cause digestive discomfort. They can be eaten boiled, roasted, barbecued, or added to soups, stuffing, sauces, desserts, and vegetable dishes. It can also be dried and ground into flour to make bread.

Chestnuts come in several varieties; Chinese variety has small sweet nuts. Malabar or Guiana variety is native to Central and South America, where it grows in swamps. Spanish variety is native to Southeast Europe and Asia Minor.

Chestnuts are relatively low in calories (195 calories/100 g) and have less fat and protein but more starch than other nuts. They are the only nuts that are rich in vitamin C. They are also rich in monounsaturated fatty acids and essential fatty acids.

Chestnuts contain fibre (8 g/100 g), B vitamins, and minerals (iron, calcium, magnesium, manganese, phosphorus, zinc, and potassium).

Because of their high starch content, chestnuts provide instant energy. Chestnuts are low in kidney-stone-forming oxalate as compared with other nuts.

CHINQUAPIN (DWARF CHESTNUT)

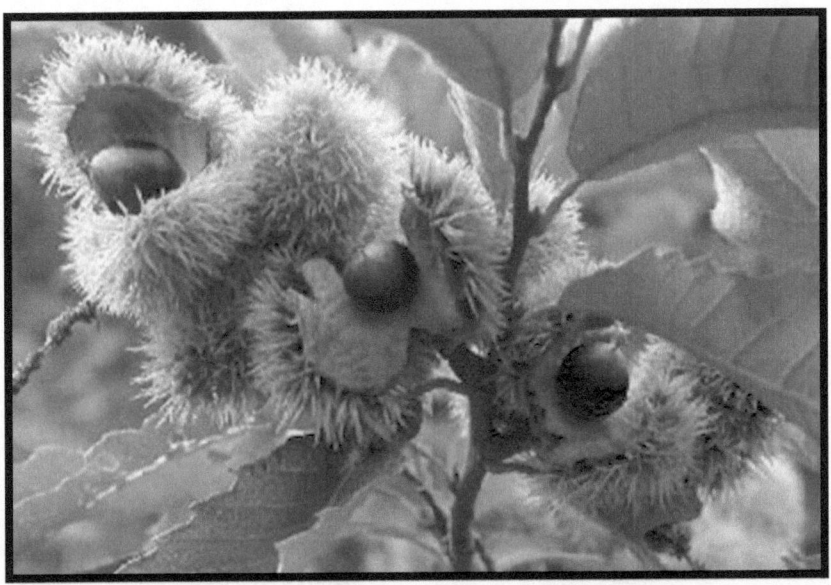

It is a small shiny brown edible, sweet chestnut-like nut, covered by a spiny tough bur. It is a small variety of the chestnut group, native to the Eastern United States.

It has a sweet nutty flavour and is loved by small mammals, like squirrels, rabbits, chipmunks, and deer mice.

Coco de mer

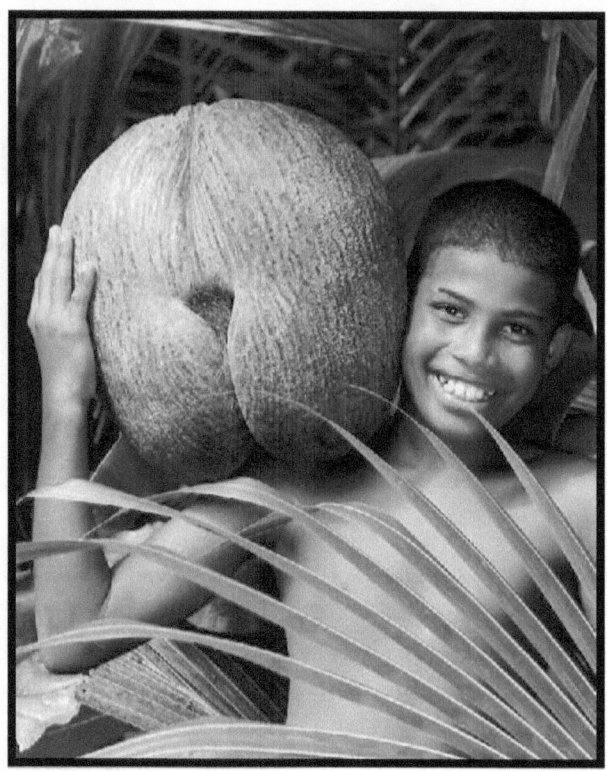

Coco de mer—also known as double coconut, sea coconut, love nut, Seychelles nut, and coco fesse—is a palm tree found only in Seychelles in the Western Indian Ocean. It is the world's largest seed, weighing as much as 42 kg, which is three times larger than regular coconut.

It is a rare and mysterious fruit, known for its rude erotic shape, resembling female buttocks. In China, the meat is used as an aphrodisiac.

The fruit is jelly-like and edible. In Chinese cuisine, it is used as a flavour enhancer. It is also used in ayurvedic and traditional Chinese medicine.

Coco de mer appears on my list of five most unusual nuts.

COCONUT (THE KING OF FOODS)

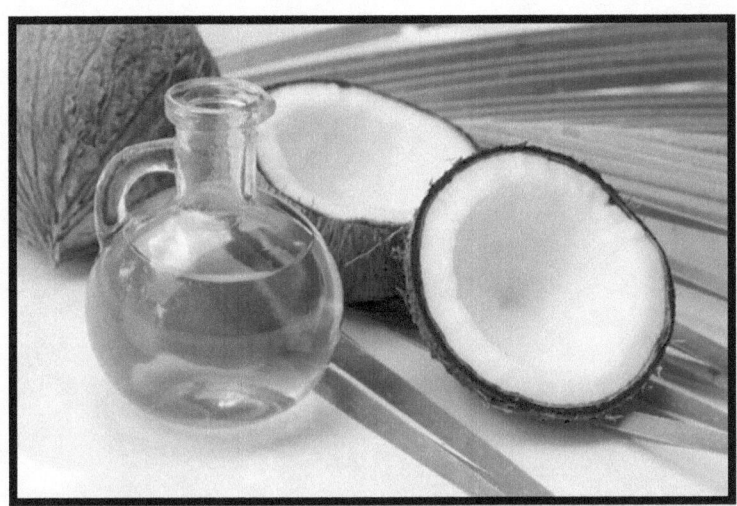

Coconut is actually not a nut but a drupe (a fleshy fruit with a central stone containing the seed). It is different from other fruits, in that it contains a large quantity of water. Coconut has been a staple food to many populations for centuries.

Coconut is rich in fibre, lauric acid (a medium-chain saturated fatty acid found in mother's milk), folic acid, manganese, copper, selenium, zinc, iron, antioxidants, enzymes, amino acids, and hormones.

Some of the health benefits of coconut meat, juice, milk, and oil are that they

1. have antimicrobial activity and boost immunity.
2. improve the heart health.
3. regulate digestion and elimination.
4. have anticancer properties, especially of colon and breast cancers.
5. rejuvenate hair and skin.
6. aid in boosting metabolism and weight loss.
7. provide quick source of energy.
8. are used for diabetics.
9. support strong bones and teeth and prevent osteoporosis.
10. coconut oil is stable at high temperature.

GINKGO NUTS

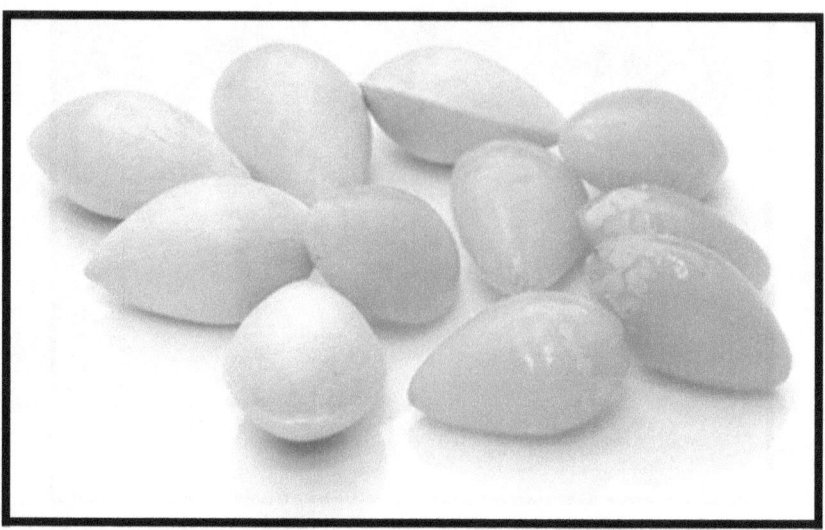

Ginkgo nuts are actually the seeds of *Ginkgo biloba* tree that originated in China millions of years ago, making it the oldest surviving tree on Earth (living fossil). It contains three coats and a kernel. After cooking, the rubbery jade-colour nut tastes like edamame (young soybean pods).

Ginkgo nut is used in Chinese traditional cuisine. For the rest of the world, it can be obtained as a supplement or tea. Ginkgo is one of the most popular supplements.

One ounce of ginkgo nut contains only 50 calories, no fat, 10 g carbohydrates, 1 g protein, and 3 g fibre. It is a good source of vitamins (A, B, and C) and minerals (iron and magnesium).

The Chinese have used the plant medicinally for a long time, but modern application is based on the German research. It is considered as a superstar herb. The nuts have similar health properties as the leaves. They have several health benefits due to their antioxidant, anti-inflammatory, antimicrobial, and vasodilatation properties.

Some of the benefits of eating gingko nuts are that they

1. enhance memory by improving blood flow to the brain.
2. enhance sexual performance by improving blood flow to the male organ.
3. suppress platelet clumping by terpenoids which dilate blood vessels.
4. contain flavonoids that serve as antioxidants, protecting the heart muscle, nerve, blood vessels, and retina from the harmful effects of free radicals.
5. help in treating vertigo, migraine, muscle cramps, and tinnitus (ringing in the ear) caused by poor blood circulation.
6. prevent asthma attacks by its anti-inflammatory action that eases swelling of the bronchial lining.
7. help in the treatment of eye disorders and hearing problems related to poor blood circulation.
8. help in the treatment of depression in the elderly.
9. boost immunity and fight infection.
10. treat urinary frequency and diarrhoea. aid in digestion. combat ageing.

Hazelnuts (Filberts)

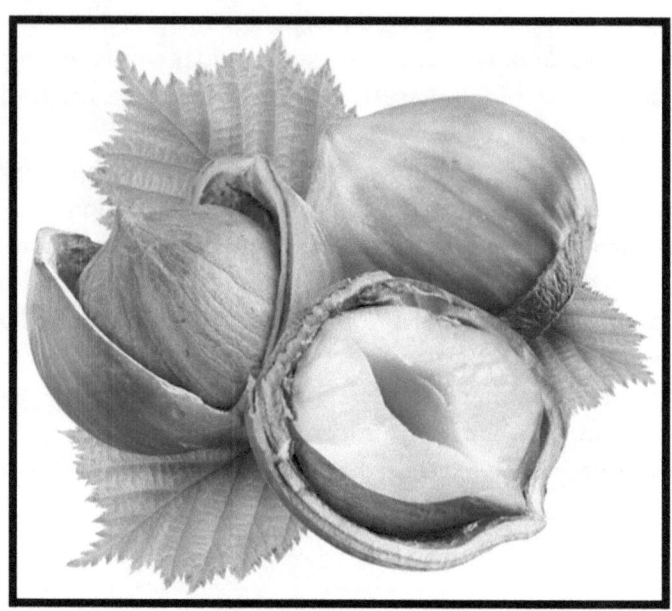

The hazel tree is a small tree originating in Turkey and Southern Europe. Hazel tree begins producing fruits three years after plantation. Turkey produces most hazelnuts, followed by Italy and the United States.

Hazelnut is sweet and is mostly used in confectionaries like biscuits, chocolates, cakes, added as a flavouring agent to coffee, or made into hazelnut butter.

One ounce of hazelnut (21 kernels) contains 178 calories, 17 g fat, and 3 g fibre. Its fat is mostly unsaturated and essential fatty acids. Hazelnut has the highest proanthocyanidin content of any tree nut that contributes to the astringent flavour and lowers the risk of blood clotting and urinary tract infection.

It contains phytosterols, powerful antioxidants that block absorption and synthesis of bad cholesterol and increases good cholesterol, thus preventing heart diseases.

It is one of the richest sources of vitamin E, the fat-soluble antioxidant that protects cell membrane from free radical damage and cuts the risk of bladder cancer by half. It also protects the skin from harmful effects of radiation, such as skin cancer and premature ageing.

It contains folic acid and vitamin B6, important for preventing heart disease. Vitamin B6 is also involved in the proper functioning of the nervous system. Folic acid is important for preventing birth defects.

It contains arginine, an amino acid that relaxes blood vessels and improves blood flow to the male organ, thus acting like Viagra.

It contains fibre, which is involved in digestive tract health. Hazelnut has many minerals such as manganese, potassium, copper, calcium, iron, magnesium, zinc, and selenium.

Hazelnut Oil

The oil has a nutty aroma and excellent astringent properties. It is a good emollient and can be used as a base oil in massages, aromatherapy, and in industries dealing with pharmaceuticals and cosmetics. It can also be used in cooking.

Kluwak Nuts

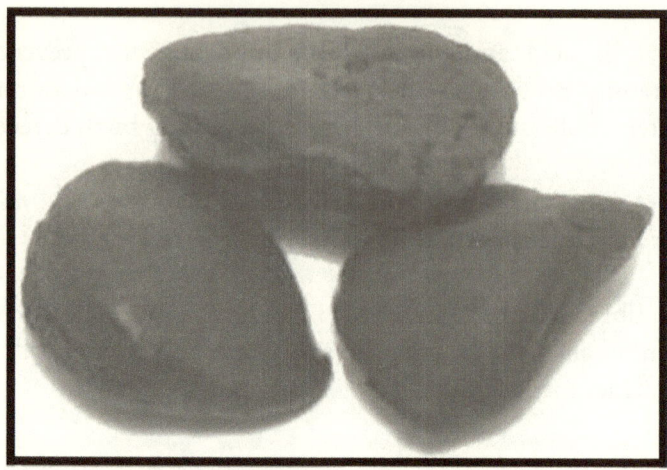

Kluwak nuts come from the kepayang tree, native to Malaysia and Indonesia. The nuts are oily and resemble Brazilian nuts in a hard black shell.

The nuts can be eaten only after boiling and fermentation to remove the toxic hydrocyanic acid. Fermented nuts become chocolate-brown, greasy, and slippery.

Cooked nuts are used in a number of popular Malaysian and Indonesian dishes.

KOLA NUT

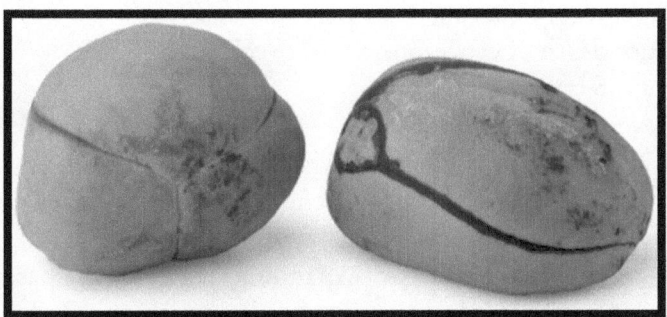

Kola nut or bitter kola is the seed kernel of a large tree (up to 18 m), native to Western and Central Africa. It was introduced to the Caribbean and Brazil by African slaves. Kola nut belongs to the cocoa family. The kola tree bears white and yellow flowers with purplish spots on them. Kola leaf is ovate shaped, pointing at both ends. The fruit is star-shaped, each producing about a dozen of square or round seeds within whitish shells.

The seeds smell like rose. The taste is initially bitter, but after chewing, it becomes sweet. The nut has to be boiled to get the kola extract. In Africa, the fresh nuts are chewed in religious rituals and are given as a gift to brides' parents and guests.

Kola nut contains caffeine (three times more than coffee), theobromine (a stimulant also found in chocolate and green tea), tannins, antioxidants (phenols and anthocyanin), sugar, starch, protein, oils, and some B vitamins.

Kola nut is not addictive and does not lead to depression.

Some of the benefits of kola nuts are that they

1. restore vitality and combat mental and physical fatigue by chewing them. They are an instant energiser.
2. stimulate the nervous system and relieve depression.

3. lead to weight loss by easing hunger pangs, decreasing food intake, suppressing appetite, and increasing metabolic rate.

4. refresh breath.

5. prevent motion sickness.

6. correct diarrhoea caused by nervousness.

7. induce death of cancerous prostate cells.

8. fight infection.

9. relieve migraine headaches.

10. aid in digestion by stimulating gastric acid secretion.

11. improve the taste of the food and are used as a flavouring agent in beverages like cola drinks.

12. act as a bronchodilator expanding the airway passages, thus relieving asthma attacks and whooping cough.

13. have a diuretic effect and rid the body of excess fluid in renal, cardiac, or rheumatic oedema.

14. relax muscles and have a calming effect.

15. boost libido and have aphrodisiac effect.

Excessive intake of kola nut, however, can lead to insomnia, anxiety, restlessness, headache, vomiting, palpitation, tremors, bone loss, and allergies like mouth ulcers. Kola nut should not be used by pregnant and lactating women.

MACADAMIA NUT

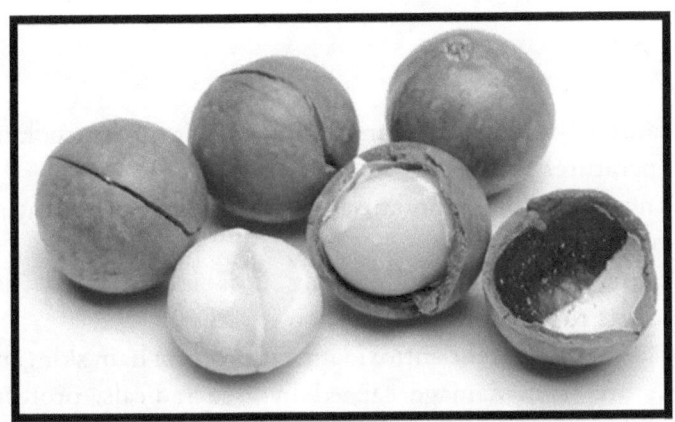

Macadamia nut is native to Australia; hence, its common name is Australian nut. It was introduced to Hawaii, New Zealand, Brazil, Indonesia, and South Africa.

The macadamia tree grows to about 15 m in height and produces fruit after seven years of plantation. Two edible species are available: smooth-shelled and rough-shelled varieties.

It has a white buttery surface and a sweet taste similar to coconut.

It is a rich source of energy (718 calories/100 g), protein (less than other nuts), fibre, phytosterols, monounsaturated fatty acids (oleic and palmitoleic acids), vitamins (A, E, and B), minerals (calcium, magnesium, manganese, iron, zinc, and selenium), simple sugars, starch, and arginine.

Some of the benefits of eating macadamia are that they have

1. potent antioxidant activities due to the presence of selenium and vitamins A and E.
2. palmitoleic acid (Omega-7 fatty acid) that curbs appetite and burns fats faster.
3. Omega-3 fatty acid that lowers the risk of heart disease and stroke.

4. arginine which is the precursor of nitric oxide, responsible for opening up blood vessels, hence aiding in erection.
5. potassium and magnesium necessary for healthy heart, muscles and nerves, water balance, and energy levels.

Macadamia Oil

1. Because of its high smoking point, it is ideal for cooking at high temperature.
2. Because of its high monounsaturated fats, it is as healthy as olive oil or canola oil.
3. Because of its high oil content, it is incorporated into beauty products to promote skin and hair health.
4. Because of its potent antioxidants, it protects hair, skin, and cellular structure from damage caused by free radicals, protects against several cancers (breast, prostate, lung, and cervix), and slows down signs of ageing.

Mamoncillo Nut

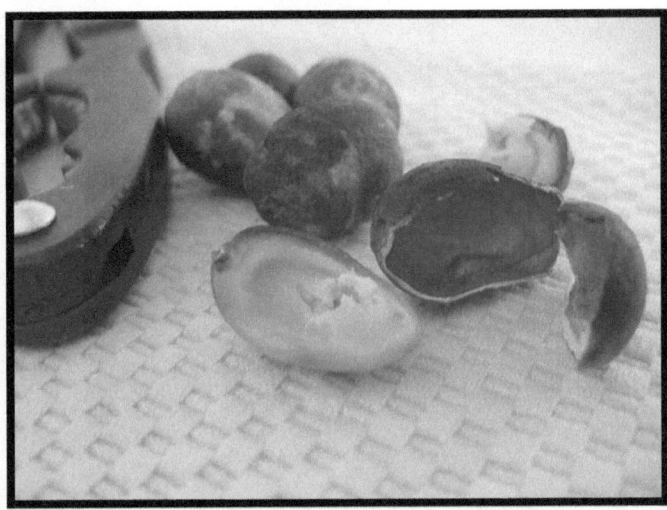

It is the seed of a Spanish lime grown in South America, Africa, and the Pacific. This fruit is related to lychee, logan, and rambutan.

The fruit is a drupe and has a thin but rigid layer of skin, enclosing a tart pulp. Most of the volume is occupied by a large seed.

The seed can be roasted like a chestnut or sesame seed, resulting in a tender nutty taste that can be eaten like sunflower seeds or chestnut. In some cultures, cooked seeds are consumed as a substitute for cassava. In Venezuela, the astringent roasted seeds are pulverised and used to treat diarrhoea.

MONGONGO NUT

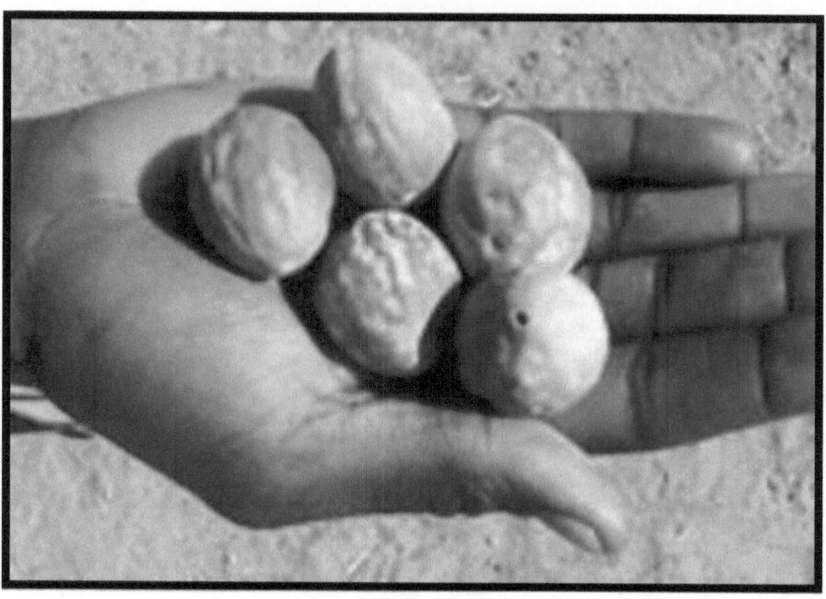

This nut is native to Southern Africa and has been a staple diet for over 7,000 years. Mongongo fruit is egg-shaped and covered with a velvety husk that contains a thin layer of edible flesh, inside of which there is a nutritive nut that can be eaten raw, roasted, or used in dishes.

Nuts are collected from elephant dung because they pass through the digestive tract of elephants intact.

The nut has 57 per cent fat (mostly unsaturated), 24 per cent protein, vitamin E, magnesium, zinc, and copper.

The pulp is red and edible and is used in preserves and porridges.

Oil obtained from the nuts can be used as skin moisturiser, conditioner, and hair and nail applications.

Mongongo nut appears on my list of five unusual nuts.

OGBONO NUT

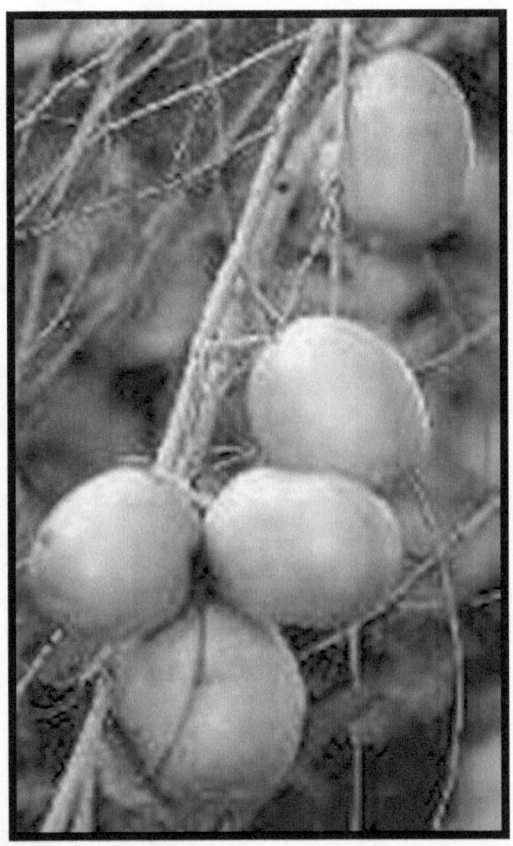

Ogbono nut is obtained from a tree native to Africa and Southeast Asia. The common names of this tree include irvingia, wild mango, African mango, bush mango, and dika. Ogbono is the Nigerian name for the kernel of the mango-like fruit. However, unlike mango, which has only one inedible seed, ogbono contains several edible seeds.

Ogbono nut is rich in fat and protein and is usually dried in the sun for preservation and is sold whole or as powder or supplement.

Because of its high mucilage content, it can be used as a thickening agent for soups and stews. The nut can also be pressed for oil that is used in cooking, as a substitute for cocoa butter, and for soap making. The pulp of the fruit is sweet and juicy and can be eaten fresh or made into preservatives and wine.

Ogbono nut lowers blood cholesterol, triglyceride, and blood pressure.

It is effective in fast weight loss by turning off appetite. Supplements of this nut are used for this purpose.

Paradise Nut (Sapucaia)

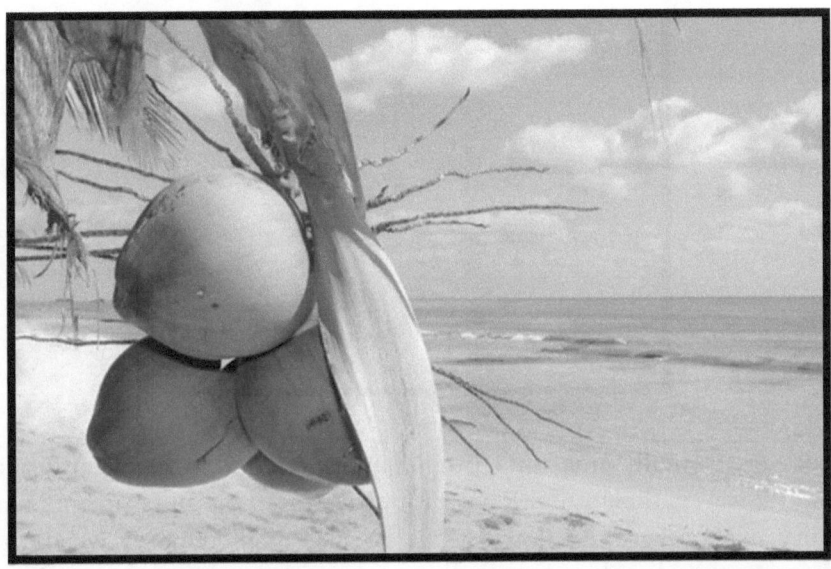

Paradise nut is called paradise because it is so delicious. It is native to the rainforests of Brazil. It belongs to the same family as the Brazil nut but is more rounded and is lighter brown in colour, has thin shells, and a softer kernel.

The tree bears coconut-sized fruits. The fruit looks like a jar with a lid and is called monkey pot because monkeys can put their paws inside the opening but cannot withdraw them after they grasp its contents. Hence, it is used as a trap for poor monkeys.

Each fruit contains 30-40 oblong-wrinkled nuts that are about two inches long.

These nuts have 61 per cent oil and 20 per cent protein. The oil is used in cooking and soap making.

PEANUTS (GROUND NUTS, EARTH NUTS)

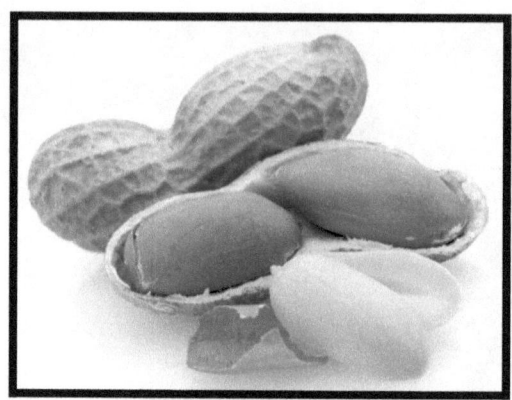

Peanuts are actually not nuts but legumes related to beans, peas, and lentils. However, their nutritional properties resemble nuts. Peanuts start growing as above-ground flowers, but because of their heavy weight after pollination, they bend and go underground, where they mature. Peanuts come in many varieties differing in size, taste, and nutritional content, but the most common varieties are the Virginia, Spanish, and Valencia.

Peanuts originated in South America, where they have existed for thousands of years. Today, the leading producers are India, China, the United States, Nigeria, and Indonesia.

Peanuts can be eaten roasted or added to desserts, confectionaries, and chutneys. Roasting enhances taste, augments the level of antioxidants like p-coumaric acid, and helps remove toxic aflatoxin. They can also be processed into a variety of forms including butter, oil, flour, and flakes.

Peanuts are rich in protein, tryptophan, arginine, fats (mainly monounsaturated), antioxidants, polyphenols, vitamin E, niacin, folic acid, copper, manganese, iron, phosphorus, magnesium, zinc, selenium, calcium, and phytosterols.

One ounce of peanuts (28 kernels) or two tablespoons of peanut butter contain 160 calories, 8 g proteins, 14 g fats, 5 g carbohydrates, and 2 g fibre.

Some of the benefits of eating peanuts are that they have

1. healthy fats that lower the risk of heart disease and diabetes.
2. high protein necessary for growth and development.
3. tryptophan that fights depression by increasing the level of serotonin in the blood.
4. arginine that increases blood flow to the male organ by changing to the vasodilator nitric oxide.
5. resveratrol that lowers the risk of cancer, heart disease, Alzheimer's disease, stroke, and infections.
6. p-coumaric acid that lowers the risk of stomach cancer by limiting the formation of carcinogenic nitrosamines in the stomach.
7. vitamin E that helps maintain the integrity of cell membrane of mucous membrane and skin by protecting from harmful free radicals.
8. beta-sitosterol that lowers risk of colon, prostate, and breast cancers.
9. fibre that helps prevent gallstones.
10. niacin that provides protection against Alzheimer's disease.
11. folic acid that prevents birth defects and maintains a healthy heart.
12. minerals that help with the formation of strong bones and teeth.

Peanut Butter

It is a paste made from ground, dry roasted peanuts, used mainly as a sandwich spread. The main producers of peanut butter are the United States and China. It has a high level of monounsaturated fats, resveratrol, vitamin E, niacin, folic acid, protein, fibre, minerals, and the antioxidant p-coumaric acid.

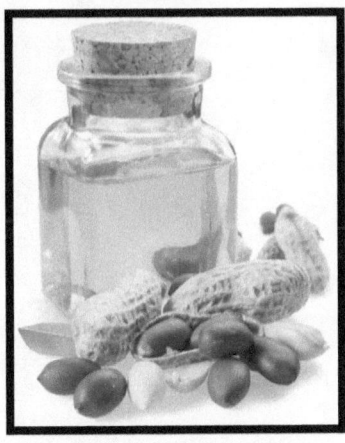

Peanut Oil

It has a pleasing taste and high smoking point, making it suitable for cooking at high temperatures like in deep-frying. It has a long shelf life. It has a very good lipid profile, having saturated, monounsaturated, and polyunsaturated fats in healthy proportions (18:49:33). Peanut oil is rich in linoleic acid (Omega-6), oleic acid, beta-sitosterol, antioxidants, vitamin E, and resveratrol. However, in animal studies, it has been shown to clog arteries.

Peanut oil can be applied directly to skin, joints, and scalp to treat eczema, arthritis, and scalp scaling, respectively. Pharmaceutical companies use peanut oil to prepare skincare products and rectal suppositories to treat constipation. Peanut oil is also used in aromatherapy and body massage.

PECAN

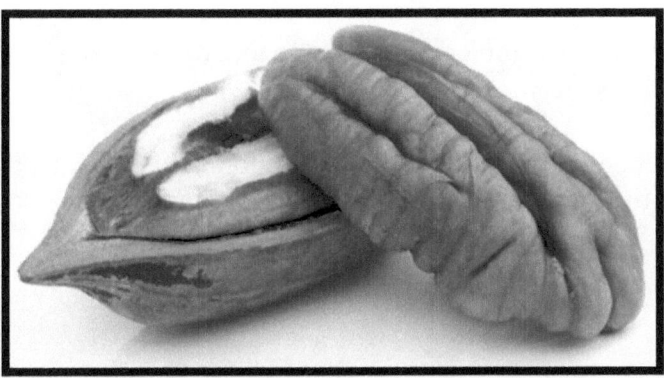

Pecan is a member of the hickory family, which also includes walnut. Pecan is the only tree nut native to North America. Up to 80 per cent of pecan is produced in the United States. The rest comes from Australia, Mexico, Brazil, Peru, China, and South Africa. The name pecan comes from the Native American word 'paccan', which means hard-shelled nut. Pecan trees can bear fruits for more than 300 years.

Pecan nut is not a true nut, but botanically, it is a drupe. Each fruit has oval to oblong shape and is dark brown in colour with a thick husk. At maturity, the husk splits off into four sections, releasing a thin-shelled nut. Nearly 1,000 varieties of pecan exist.

Pecan is sweet, buttery and can be eaten on its own or added to desserts and confectionaries and made into pecan butter.

Pecan is nutrient-dense, rich in vitamins (E, A, and B), minerals (manganese, copper, zinc, phosphorus, iron, magnesium, calcium, and selenium), healthy fats, protein, fibre, sterols, and antioxidants. A 1 oz serving (20 halves) contains 196 calories, 20 g fat (mostly unsaturated), and 2.7 g fibre. Pecans rank highest among all nuts in antioxidant levels. It contains ellagic acid, vitamin E, and carotenoids that work synergistically to remove toxic free radicals, thus protecting the body from heart diseases, cancers, Alzheimer's disease, and infections.

Phytosterols hinder absorption of cholesterol from the gut, leading to lower blood cholesterol, thus lowering the risk of heart diseases.

Beta-sitosterol lowers the risk of an enlarged prostate.

Pecans may aid in weight loss and maintenance by increasing metabolic rate and enhancing satiety.

Gamma-tocopherol, the form of vitamin E found in pecan, has been found to kill the prostate cancer cells.

Vitamin B acts as cofactors in enzymatic reactions in the body.

Pecan Oil

It has a mild nutty flavour and is ideal for cooking at high temperatures. It is also used in salad dressing, aromatherapy, and cosmetics.

PEKEA NUT

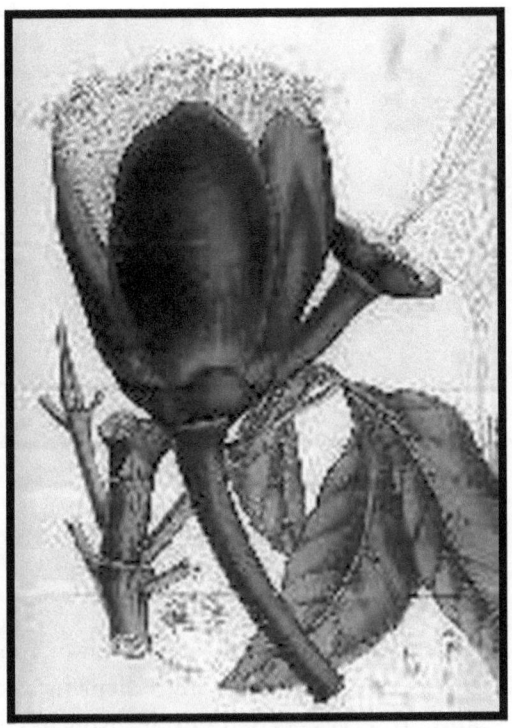

Pekea nut, also known as souari nut and butternut, is native to South America. Its coconut-sized fruit has four nuts surrounded by an edible flesh. The warty red hard-shelled, kidney-shaped edible nuts have a rich flavour and are used as food and as a source of cooking oil.

Pili Nuts

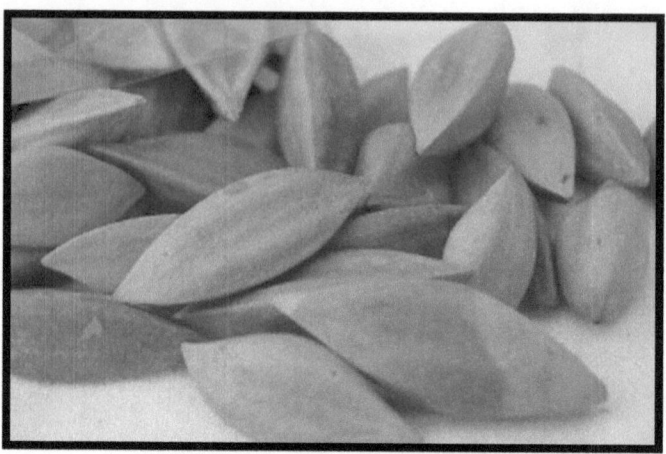

Pili nut is native to the Philippines. The light-brown triangular nut is enclosed in a rough thick dark shell. The shell must be removed before eating the nut because it causes diarrhoea.

Pili nut is crispy and delicious. It can be eaten fresh or roasted and used in cooking or in salads. It is also used as an ingredient in cakes, puddings, ice creams, chocolates, and preserves. When raw, it tastes like roasted pumpkin seeds, and when roasted, it tastes like almonds.

Pili nuts are rich in fibre, protein, monounsaturated fats, vitamins E and B, magnesium, copper, and manganese. It contains 71 per cent fat, 11 per cent protein, and 8 per cent carbohydrates.

The kernel is used as a laxative.

Emulsion from crushed kernels is used as a substitute for infants' milk and for making medicinal ointments.

The fruit pulp and the young shoots are used to make pickles, flour, sauce, or a puree.

Pili oil is used in cooking, lamp oil, soaps, cosmetics, and pharmaceutical products.

Pine Nuts

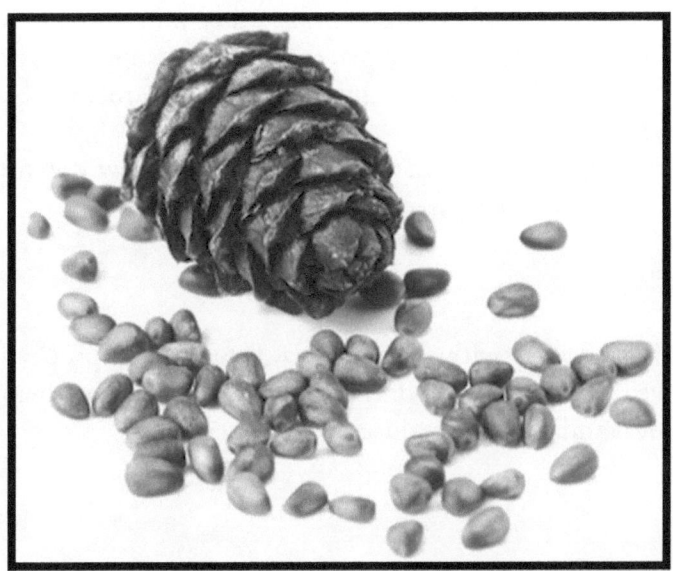

Pine nuts are botanically not nuts but are the seeds of about twenty different species of pine cones. Pine trees grow in wild forest regions of the northern hemisphere, especially in Siberia and Canada. The flowers of the pine tree develop into a cone. Once mature and dry, the cones open up and release the seeds. The seeds are elongated, ivory-coloured, half an inch long, with a soft texture and sweet buttery flavour.

Pine nuts are used as a salad topper in pasta and in desserts.

Pine nuts are rich in antioxidants, phytosterols, vitamins (A, E, K, and niacin), minerals (zinc, phosphorus, iron, copper, manganese, magnesium, and potassium), fibre, protein, calories (673 calories/100 g), and monounsaturated fatty acids.

Some of the benefits of eating pine nuts include the following:

1. Weight loss: although pine nuts are high in fats, eating pine nuts causes weight loss because they contain pinoleic acid that suppresses the appetite by triggering the release of hunger-suppressing

hormones CCK (cholecystokinin) and glp-1 (glucagon-like peptide-1) in the gut.

2. Cardiovascular support: they contain monounsaturated fatty acids like oleic acid that lowers bad cholesterol, thus lowering the risk of heart attack. They also contain other nutrients like vitamin E, vitamin K, manganese, copper, and iron that support heart health.

3. Eye health: they contain lutein and beta-carotene that support heart health.

4. Anti-ageing: they contain antioxidants that slow down the ageing process by removing free radicals from the body.

Pine Nut Oil

It has a delicate flavour with sweet aroma. Its emollient properties help to keep skin well protected from dryness. It is used in aromatherapy and in pharmaceutical and cosmetic industries.

PISTACHIOS

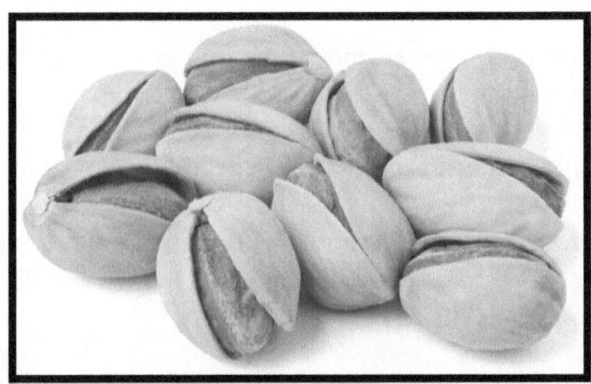

Pistachio is a member of the cashew family. It originated in West Asia and is now produced in large scale in Iran, the United States, Syria, Turkey, and China. It has been cultivated for over 10,000 years. It is mentioned, along with almonds, in the Old Testament. The name pistachio is the Italian version of the Persian word 'pistah', meaning nut. In Iran, it is called the 'smiling pistachio', and in China, it is called the 'happy nut'. After plantation, it takes eight years to produce nuts, bearing fruits for centuries.

The fruit is a drupe (a fruit with a large single edible seed). The tree bears heavy clusters of fruits like grape bunches.

The mature fruit has an off-white hard shell that splits exposing a green oblong kernel, which has a sweet taste and fruity aroma. Pistachio differs from all other nuts, in that it is green in colour and has a semi-opened shell.

Pistachio can be eaten on its own or added to salads, cakes, biscuits, and chocolates.

Pistachio is rich in vitamins (B, A, E, and C), minerals (copper, phosphorus, manganese, magnesium, potassium, calcium, selenium, and zinc), fibre, protein, monounsaturated fatty acid like oleic acid, sterols, and antioxidants.

A 1 oz serving of pistachios (50 kernels) provides 150 calories, 13 g fat, and 3 g fibre.

Pistachio is called skinny nut because each nut has only 3 calories. The potassium content of pistachios is more than most other nuts.

Some of the benefits of eating pistachios include the following:

Heart health: its high antioxidants and monounsaturated fatty acid fight inflammation, protecting blood vessels and lowering the risk of heart diseases.

Eye health: its carotenoids protect the eye from free radical damage.

Skin health: vitamin E maintains the integrity of cell membranes in the skin. It also protects the skin from UV damage, defending against premature ageing and skin cancer.

Nervous system health: vitamin B6 helps to create the myelin insulating sheath around nerve fibres that allows optimal messaging between nerves. B6 is also involved in the synthesis of melatonin, serotonin, epinephrine, and GABA F (an amino acid that calms transmission of nerve impulses in the nervous system).

Blood: vitamin B6, folic acid, iron, and copper are important for haemoglobin production.

Immunity: vitamin B6 maintains the health of spleen, lymph nodes, and thymus, ensuring the production of white blood cells that defend the body from infection.

Diabetes: the special antioxidants found in pistachios can prevent the harmful process of glycation (bonding of protein molecule with sugar molecule), which makes proteins unusable, ultimately helping diabetes to damage tissues as sugars end up bonding inappropriately.

Pistachio Oil

The oil is flavourful and has a pleasant nutty aroma. It has excellent emollient properties. It keeps skin well protected from dryness. It is used in cooking and as base oil in massage therapy, aromatherapy, and in pharmaceutical and cosmetic industries.

SOY NUTS

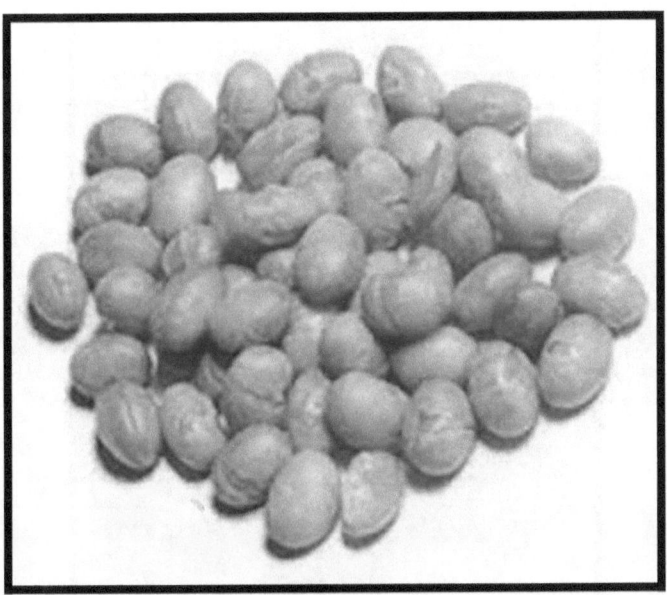

Soy nuts are made from soybeans, which have been soaked in water, drained, and then roasted or baked until brown and crispy. Soy nuts are similar in texture and flavour to peanuts and can be eaten as nuts or covered with seasonings, honey, chocolate, or yogurt.

Some of the health benefits of eating soy nuts are that they are

1. rich in high-quality protein (75 per cent) similar to animal proteins.
2. rich in Omega-3 fatty acids that prevent cardiovascular diseases.
3. rich in fibre that aid in weight reduction if eaten in moderation.
4. rich in magnesium and potassium that aid in lowering blood pressure.
5. rich in isoflavones that lower signs of ageing and menopausal symptoms and prevent osteoporosis and prostate cancer.

Tiger Nut (Earth Almond)

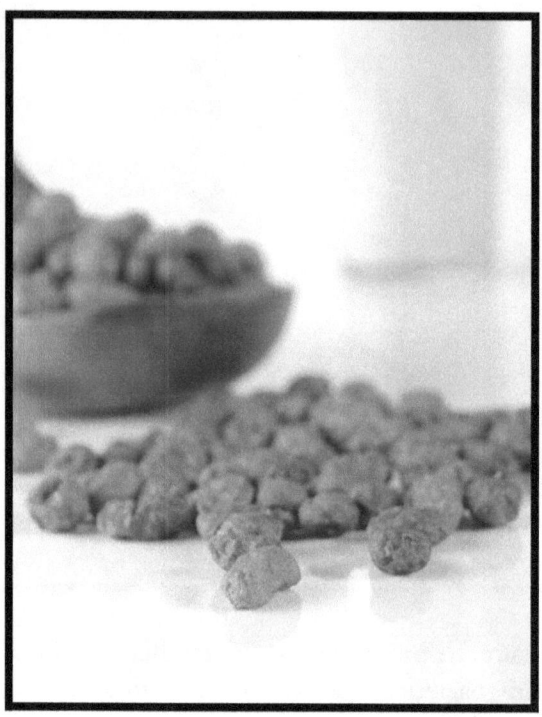

Tiger nuts were cultivated by the Egyptians more than 4,000 years ago. It is native to the Mediterranean region and is widely used in Spain, where it is known as 'chufa'. Tiger nut is actually not a nut but a small tuber that grows like weeds and provides good nutrients cheaply.

It tastes like a crunchy caramel and comes in many sizes and colours (brown, black, and yellow).

It can be eaten raw, roasted, dried or baked or processed into milk, flour, and oil. It is used as a flavouring agent in ice cream and biscuits.

It is rich in fibre, protein, essential amino acids, sugars, oleic acid, vitamins (E, C, and B), and minerals (potassium, calcium, phosphorus, magnesium, and manganese).

Tiger nut oil is considered a healthy alternative to olive oil. It is used in cooking and in pharmaceutical and cosmetic industries.

Some of the benefits of eating tiger nuts are that they

1. are a good source of energy.
2. aid in digestion by providing digestive enzymes and relieve flatulence.
3. increase blood circulation.
4. lower cholesterol and hardening of arteries.
5. decrease pain from arthritis. relieve gum ulcer.
6. stimulate the immune system.
7. aid in treating diarrhoea.
8. increase sexual performance.
9. liberate the hormone that produces insulin, thus useful for diabetics.

Walnuts (The King of Nuts)

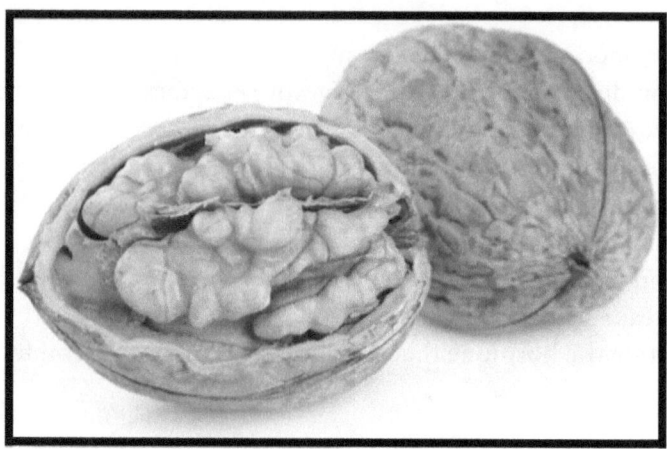

Native to Persia, walnuts are also commercially produced in California, Turkey, China, France, and Romania. After plantation, the tree takes four years to produce fruits, and it produces for forty-five years. The Greeks called it 'the nut of Jupiter', the nut for the gods.

Walnut kernel consists of two partially attached bumpy lobes that are off-white in colour and covered by a thin light-brown skin. Walnuts have been regarded as the symbol of intellectuals because the kernels resemble brain.

Walnuts can be eaten raw or added to yogurt, pizzas, salads, desserts, and confectionaries.

Walnuts are rich sources of fibre, protein, healthy fats, vitamins (E and B), minerals (manganese, copper, potassium, calcium, phosphorus, iron, magnesium, zinc, and selenium), and phytochemicals. One ounce (14 halves) contains 185 calories, 18 g fat, and 2 g fibre.

Some of the benefits of eating walnuts are that they

1. contain high oleic acid and Omega-3 fatty acids that lower bad cholesterol, thus decreasing blood pressure, heart diseases, and stroke. Only a handful of walnuts contain as much Omega-3 as 3

oz of salmon. They are the only nuts with alpha-linolenic (ALA) as Omega-3 fatty acid.

2. have the highest level of phytochemical antioxidants, such as melatonin, ellagic acids, vitamin E, carotenoids, and polyphenolic compounds among all other nuts. They help against cancer, ageing, inflammation, and neurological diseases.

3. are an excellent source of vitamin E, which is required for maintaining the integrity of cell membranes of mucus and skin by protecting them from harmful free radicals.

4. have melatonin that regulates sleep and light-dark adjustments.

5. have arginine which is converted to nitric oxide, a vasodilator that increases blood flow to the male organ, improving its sexual performance.

6. improve sperm quality (vitality, mobility, and morphology).

7. have B vitamins which make it an ideal nut during pregnancy.

8. have biotin that strengthens hair texture, improves hair growth, and decreases hair fall.

9. have a positive impact on diabetics.

10. can be included in weight management programmes if eaten in moderation.

11. improve bone strength.

Walnut Oil

It has a flavourful nutty aroma and astringent properties. It is used in cooking and locally to protect skin from dryness and as a carrier in massage therapy, aromatherapy, and in the pharmaceutical and cosmetic industries.

Varieties of Walnuts

There are more than thirty varieties of walnuts. The most popular are

1. Persian or English or common walnut: this variety has a thin shell which is easily cracked. The curly nutmeat halves have a sweet flavour.

2. Black walnut: it is native to America. Its hard sticky shells protect dark-skinned white nutmeat. Its rich nutty flavour is superior to other varieties when used in confectionaries and baked products,

but it is not recommended as snack because its flavour is disagreeable.

3. White walnut or butternut: it is native to the Eastern United States and Southeast Canada. It is the hardiest member of the walnut family.

4. Japanese walnut or heart nut: it is native to Japan, and the kernel is shaped like a heart. It is easy to crack. It has a sweet buttery taste because of its high oil content.

5. Red walnut: it is a hybrid of the Persian red-skinned walnut and the creamy English walnut, creating an amazing taste. The nut is red only on the outside with the creamy white flesh inside.

TOP FIVE HEALTHIEST NUTS

Almonds   Pistachios
Hazelnuts   Walnuts
Pecans

Five Most Unusual Nuts

Bat nut

Barking deer's mango nut

Candlenut

Coco de mer

Mongongo nut

Top Ten Most Produced Nuts

Coconuts   Chestnuts

Peanuts   Betel nuts

Cashew nuts Hazelnuts

Almonds   Pistachios

Walnuts   Kola nuts

SEEDS

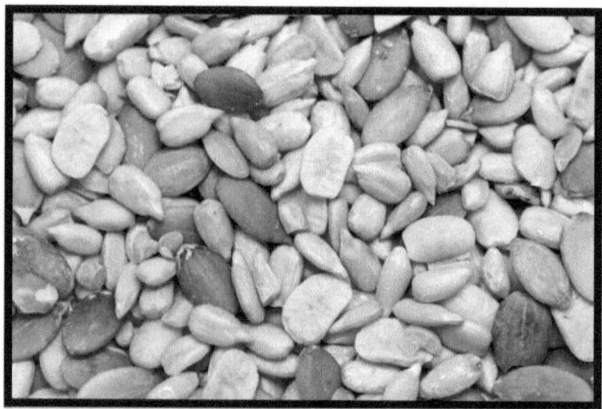

Eating seeds regularly is a good habit. Not only do they taste good but are also good sources of antioxidants, phytosterols, fibre, protein, essential amino acids, monounsaturated fatty acids, Omega fatty acids, vitamins, and minerals essential for healthy body and mind.

Some of the benefits of eating seeds are that they

1. are quick natural source of energy.
2. may prevent heart diseases.
3. may prevent certain cancers.
4. may prevent inflammations like rheumatism and asthma.
5. may prevent nervous disorders like Alzheimer's disease and parkinsonism.
6. may prevent osteoporosis.
7. may boost immunity and prevent infection.
8. may aid in controlling blood sugar.
9. may support weight loss.
10. may normalise and regulate bowel movement.

A serving size for seeds is 1 oz or 28 g, equivalent to three tablespoons.

ALPHABETICAL LIST OF SEEDS

Black Seed
Canola Seed
Chia Seed
Colocynth Seed
Drupe Seeds
Flaxseed
Grape Seed
Hemp Seed
Jackfruit Seed
Kiwi Seed

Melon Seed
Perilla Seed
Poppy Seed
Pumpkin Seed
Quinoa Seed
Safflower Seed
Sesame Seed
Sunflower Seed
Watermelon Seed

List of Seed Families

Composite family: Sunflower seed
Flax family: Flaxseed
Gourd family: Pumpkin seed
Pedalium family: Sesame seed
Poppy family: Poppy seed

BLACK SEEDS (BLACK CUMIN)

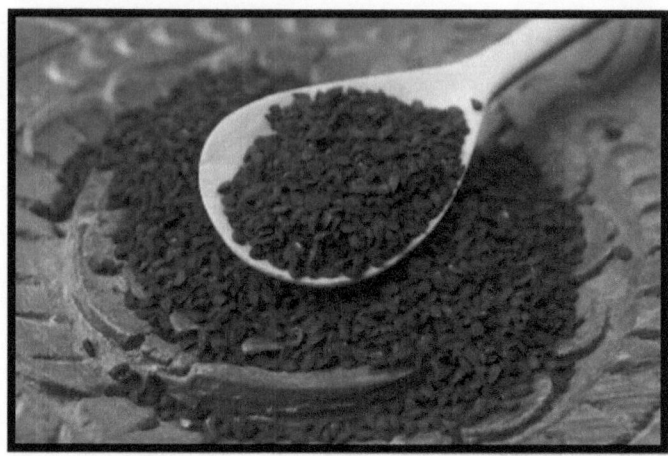

In Arabic it is known as 'habbatul barakah', meaning seed of blessing. It originated in Egypt. Black seed oil was found in Egyptian Pharaoh Tutankhamun's tomb 3,300 years ago. For centuries, black seed and its oil have been used by millions of people in India, Middle East, and the Mediterranean for medicinal purposes. Today, it is used as a seasoning spice due to its nutty flavour across the world.

The Prophet Mohammed declared it as 'a remedy for all diseases except death'.

Black seed is an aromatic spice, similar in size to sesame seeds, and is crescent-shaped. It grows in a small pod, and in order to get to it, water must be poured over it. It can be consumed in salads, soups, and with yogurts or pressed for its oil.

Black seeds contain more than 100 valuable nutrients, including Omega-3 fatty acids, beta-sitosterol, saponins, alkaloids, fibre, protein, vitamins (B, A, and C), and minerals (calcium, iron, copper, zinc, phosphorus, potassium, magnesium, and selenium).

Some of the benefits of eating black seeds are that they

1. boost the immune system and fight infections.
2. decrease allergic reactions.
3. fight some cancers like that of the colon and pancreas.
4. treat gastrointestinal problems like flatulence, diarrhoea, dysentery, constipation, and haemorrhoids.
5. treat respiratory conditions like asthma, cough, and flu symptoms.
6. treat skin conditions like eczema, acne, psoriasis, and boils.
7. protect liver and kidney.
8. treat pink eyes (conjunctivitis).
9. start menses and increase milk flow in nursing mothers.
10. have analgesic effect and decrease joint pain, headache, and toothache.
11. protect heart by lowering cholesterol and blood pressure.
12. stimulate energy production and help recovery from fatigue.
13. are beneficial for type 2 diabetes by inhibiting glucose synthesis and sensitising insulin.

Canola Seeds (Rapeseed Oil)

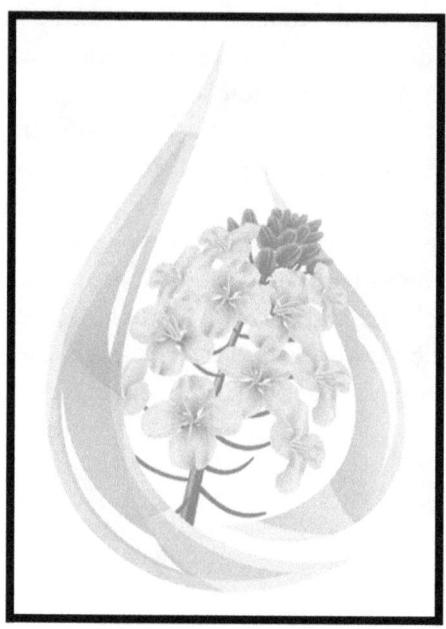

Canola seeds belong to the Brassica family, which also includes mustard, turnip, Brussels sprouts, cabbage, kale, cauliflower, broccoli, and so on.

Each seed pod contains 20-35 tiny rods, mustard-like seeds that contain 40 per cent oil. Canola or rapeseed oil is light yellow in colour and has a neutral taste. It has a high smoking point, making it ideal for cooking at high temperatures, like in deep-frying. It is a stable cooking oil having a very long shelf life. It is also used in salad dressing, margarines, spreads, and baking.

Canola oil is high in energy (884 calories/100 g). However, its high ratio of monounsaturated fats to saturated fats makes it healthy oil. It has twice the Omega-3 fatty acid present in olive oil. It also contains vitamin E and plant sterols.

Canola oil reduces symptoms of diseases associated with inflammatory processes like arthritis, heart diseases, Alzheimer's disease, and certain cancers.

Chia Seeds

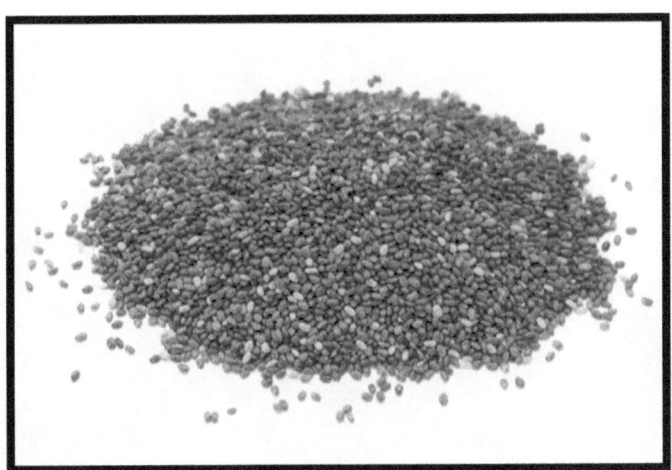

Chia belongs to the mint family. Chia is native to Central and South America. Chia is the Maya word for strength.

Chia seeds are tiny 1 mm oval mottled-coloured with brown, grey, black, and white seeds that have a mild flavour. They can be eaten raw, sprinkled on cereals, sauces, vegetables, rice dishes, and yogurt, or mixed into drinks and baked products. They can also be mixed with water and made into a gel. The mild nutty flavour of chia seeds make them easy to add to foods and beverages.

One ounce (28 g or 2 tablespoons) of chia seeds contains 9 g fat, 4 g protein, 11 g fibre, 12 g carbohydrates, besides calcium, phosphorus, and manganese.

Some of the benefits of chia seeds are that they

1. are the richest sources of Omega-3 fatty acids that protect against inflammatory diseases like asthma, heart diseases, arthritis, and certain cancers.
2. lower blood pressure.
3. create a sense of fullness because they absorb water and form a bulky gel.

75

4. can be used by athletes for hydration and endurance.
5. aid in intestinal regularity.
6. control blood glucose level by slowing down the conversion of complex carbohydrates to simple sugars.

COLOCYNTH SEEDS

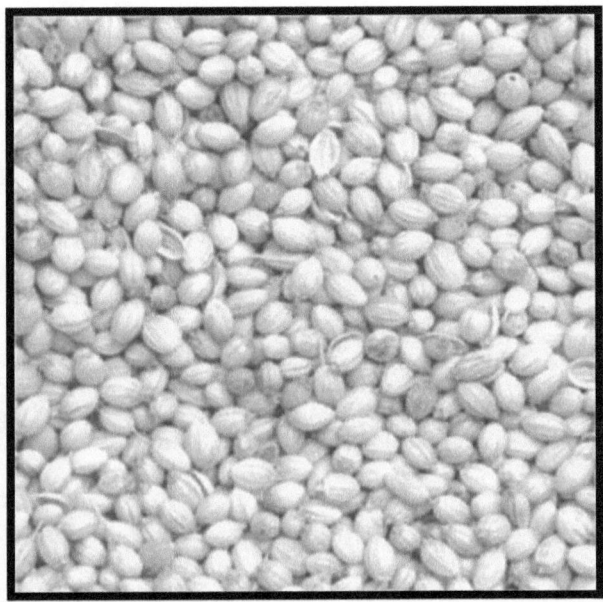

Colocynth is a relative of the watermelon and is native to tropical Africa and Asia. Colocynth is also known as bitter apple, bitter cucumber, and desert gourd. It is a desert vine plant that resembles the common watermelon but bears small hard fruits with a bitter pulp.

The seeds are small (about 6 mm), smooth brown when ripe, ovoid-shaped and edible but bitter with a nutty flavour. The seeds are rich in oil, protein, tryptophan, arginine, sulphur-containing amino acids, calcium, and niacin. Colocynth seeds improve digestion and strengthen immunity.

DRUPE SEEDS

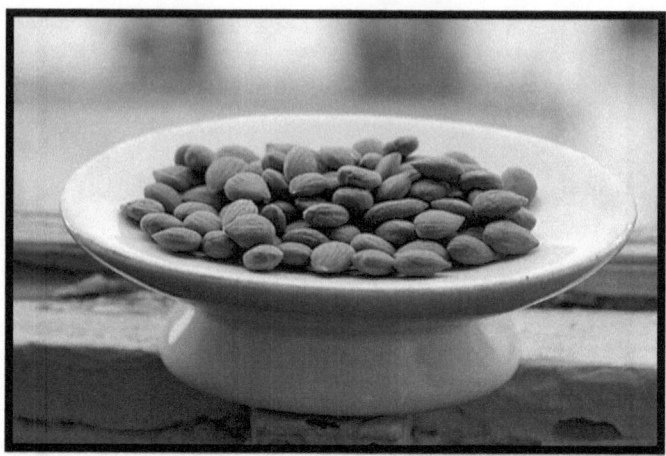

Drupe is a fruit in which an outer fleshy pulp surrounds a stony pit with a single seed (kernel) inside. Such drupes include apricot, peach, nectarine plum, and cherry.

Drupe seeds are good sources of the bitter amygdalin, also known as laetrile, and vitamin B17, which is actually not a vitamin but a cyanogenic glycoside. Glycoside is a compound in which a bond has formed between glucose and another nutrient. In this case, this other nutrient is the toxic cyanide. In the body, amygdalin is converted to cyanide, which is poisonous and can cause serious side effects, including death.

It is the cyanide constituent that destroys the cancerous cells. The body can detoxify a small portion of cyanide, but eating too many seeds containing amygdalin maybe hazardous to health. The more bitter the taste, the higher content of cyanide and greater the risk.

In Chinese medicine, laetrile is used to combat cancer, stimulate respiration, improve digestion, decrease blood pressure, and lower arthritic pain.

B17 is available as a supplement in cancer clinics outside the United States.

FLAXSEEDS (LINSEEDS)

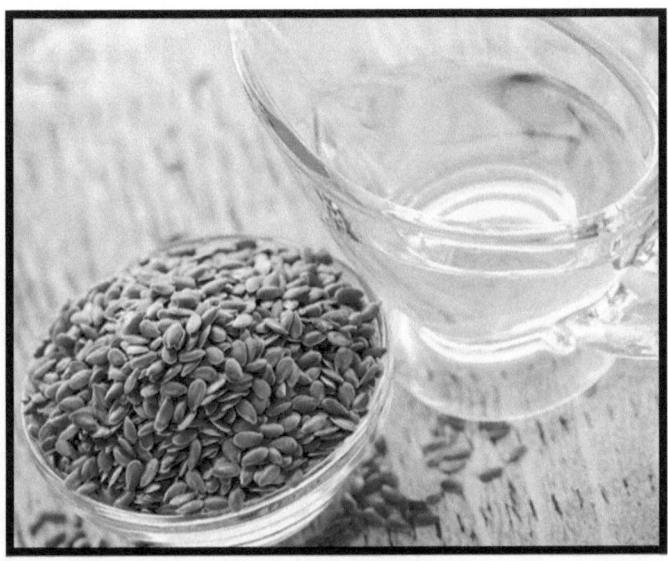

Flaxseed is native to the Middle East and India. It was cultivated in Babylon around 3000 BC. The ancient Egyptians used it as food and medicine. Now, it grows in Canada and the Northern United States.

Flaxseed is a blue-flowered herb with brown or golden-yellow seeds. There are hundreds of flax-based products like crackers, waffles, and oatmeal available in the markets.

Flaxseed is rich in Omega-3 fatty acids, lignans, fibre, protein, tryptophan, manganese, magnesium, phosphorus, copper, and thiamine. They contain Omega-3 fatty acids that have anti-inflammatory action, thus lowering arthritic pain, asthma, heart diseases, and certain cancers. High fibre and mucilage content make it a good laxative, lower bad cholesterol, and stabilise blood glucose.

Flaxseeds are the best source of lignans in our diet. Lignans have both plant oestrogen and antioxidant properties. They promote fertility, decrease premenstrual symptoms (bloating and pain) and postmenopausal symptoms (hot flashes, mood disturbances, and dryness of vagina), and prevent some cancers (breast, prostate, and colon).

Tryptophan boosts mood and alleviates depression.

Flaxseed oil has a flavourful nutty aroma and is used as carrier in traditional medicine and pharmaceutical industries.

GRAPE SEEDS

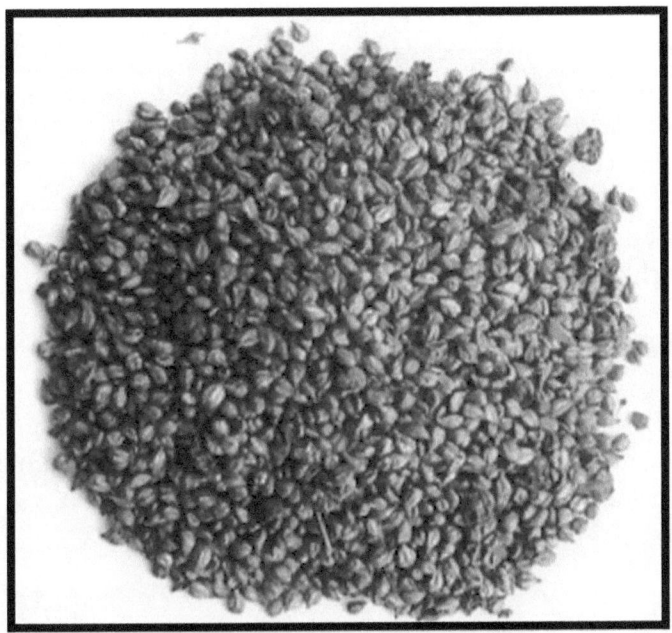

You may be surprised to learn that grape seed extract (GSE) could be more beneficial than the grape itself. So, eat your grapes with their seeds and do not seek seedless grapes.

GSE is rich in procyanidin, the antioxidant which has fifty times more than vitamin C in fighting free radicals. Other antioxidants found in GSE are vitamin E, essential fatty acids, flavonoids, and resveratrol.

Thanks to those powerful antioxidants; GSE has anti-inflammatory, anti-ageing, anti-cancerous, antimicrobial, anti-allergic, and immune-boosting properties.

Some of the benefits of GSE are that it

1. lowers blood pressure and heart diseases.
2. provides treatment for poor blood circulation like varicose veins and haemorrhoids.

3. treats the swelling caused by injury or surgery or arthritis.
4. helps with eye diseases related to diabetes.
5. treats skin diseases like dermatitis, acne, wrinkles, dry itching skin, age spots, sunburn, chipped lips, wounds, bruising, and stretch marks.
6. decreases premenstrual symptoms.
7. treats hair loss and dandruff.
8. helps in weight loss.
9. decreases risk of colorectal cancer.
10. has a neuroprotective property.

A word of caution for those taking blood thinners like warfarin: it might interfere with anticoagulation, hence causing excessive bleeding.

Grape Seed Oil

This oil is used in cooking, salad dressings, confectionaries, skin moisturisers, aromatherapy, massage therapy, hair products, sunblocks, and sunburn ointments.

HEMP SEEDS

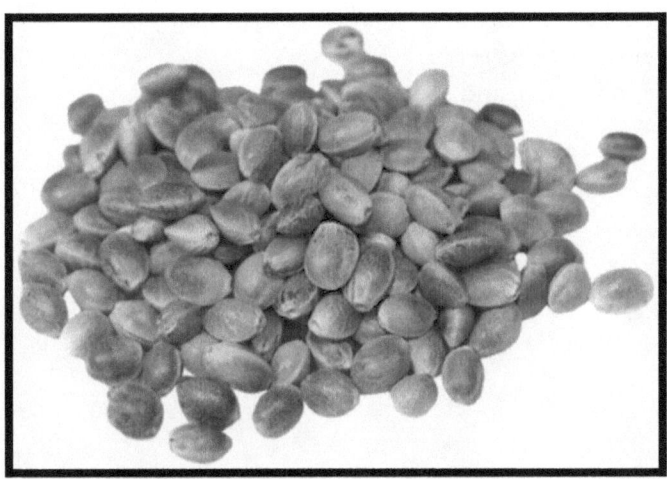

Hemp—also known as cannabis, marijuana, and qunnab—is one of the earliest domesticated plants cultivated by many civilisations for more than 12,000 years. Hemp oil is mentioned in the Bible. Today, China is the main producer of hemp.

Hemp seed has 44 per cent edible oil, 80 per cent of which is essential fatty acids, 33 per cent complete protein, 6 per cent fibre, calories (587 calories/100 g), vitamin E, magnesium, zinc, potassium, iron, calcium, phosphorus, copper, and manganese.

Hemp seeds are the most nutritious seeds in the world and are the only food source that contains all the essential amino acids and all the essential fatty acids. They have a mild nutty flavour and can be eaten raw, ground, made into milk, prepared as tea, and used in baking.

Some of the benefits of hemp seeds are that they

1. lower cholesterol and blood pressure and improve cardiovascular health.
2. boost immunity.
3. lower premenstrual symptoms.

4. decrease inflammation and symptoms from arthritis.
5. improve skin and hair condition.
6. increase energy level.
7. may help promote learning and memory by stimulating the brain enzyme calcineurin.
8. lower the risk of certain cancers.
9. act as a laxative and treat constipation.

JACKFRUIT SEEDS

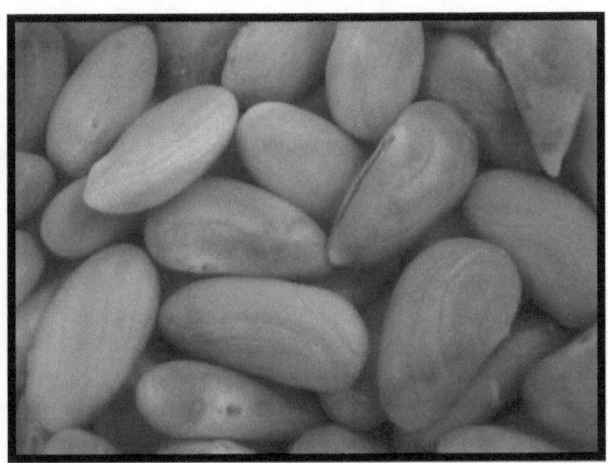

Jackfruit nuts are the seeds or pods that are enclosed in the sweet yellow flesh of the jackfruit.

Seeds can be boiled, roasted, fried or dried, and ground into flour. Their taste and texture are similar to those of the chestnut.

The seeds are round and dark and are commonly found in Southeast Asia. They contain 38 per cent carbohydrates, 6.6 per cent protein, 14 per cent fat, fibre, vitamins (B, A, and C), minerals (calcium, phosphorus, and zinc), lignans, isoflavones, and saponins.

Jackfruit seeds have many health benefits like anti-ulcer, anticancer, antihypertensive, anti-ageing, and antioxidant properties.

KIWI SEEDS

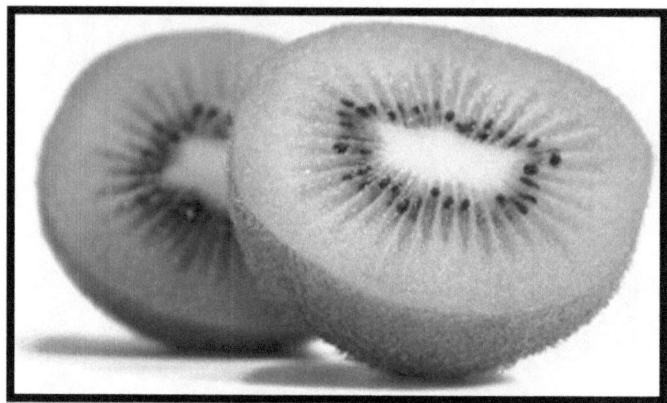

Kiwi seeds are tiny black seeds that constitute less than 3 per cent of the weight of the kiwi. They have high nutrient content and store the essential nutrients for the growth of new plant. They are rich in alpha-linolenic acid (ALA), which is an important Omega-3 fatty acid that helps in the development of the brain and protects the heart.

Kiwi seed oil contains vitamin A and is used in skin and haircare products. Kiwi seed oil can be purchased as a supplement.

Melon Seeds

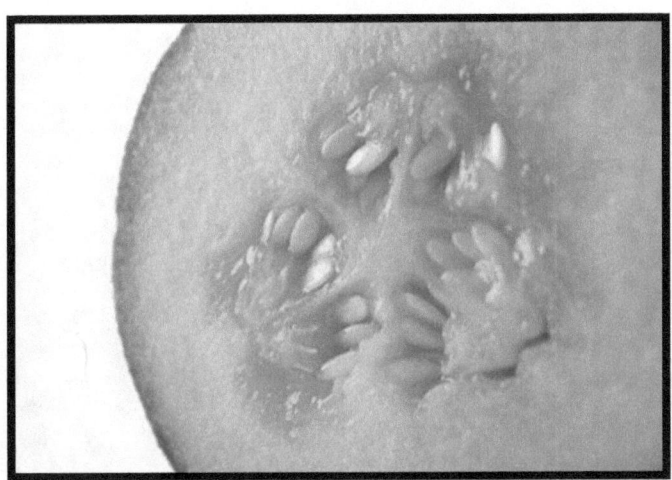

Melon originated in Africa, Middle East, and Southwest Asia thousands of years ago.

Melon seed has a greyish white hard shell with a white inner kernel that has a sweet nutty flavour. They are used as snacks after roasting, in baking and confectionary, sweets, and refreshing drinks.

Melon seeds contain Omega-3 fatty acids, protein, vitamin B, zinc, potassium, manganese, magnesium, iron, copper, and calcium.

Some of the benefits of melon seeds are that they

1. help lower cholesterol and protect the heart.
2. aid in intestinal regularity.
3. aid in weight loss.
4. help in skin and hair disorders.
5. help in nervous disorders.
6. boost the immune system.

Perilla (Shizo) Seeds (Wild Sesame)

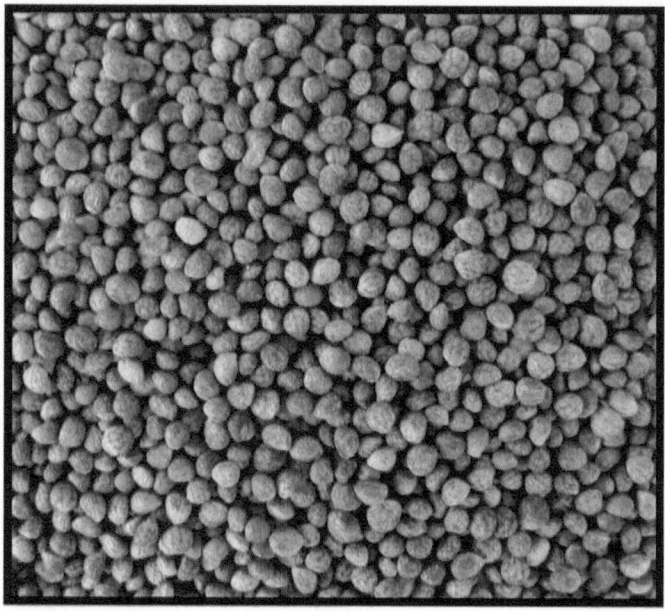

Perilla seeds come from the perilla herb, native to the mountains of East Asia. It belongs to the mint family. The perilla plant is edible and medicinal.

The seeds are tiny 1 mm in size and oval-shaped. Externally, the seeds are greyish-brown with purple lines, and internally, they are yellowish white. The taste is mild and can be eaten raw or finely ground into powder.

Perilla seeds are nutritive powerhouses, containing Omega-3 fatty acids, amino acids, vitamins, minerals, and fibre. In Chinese medicine, perilla seeds are used for the treatment of asthma and constipation.

POPPY SEEDS

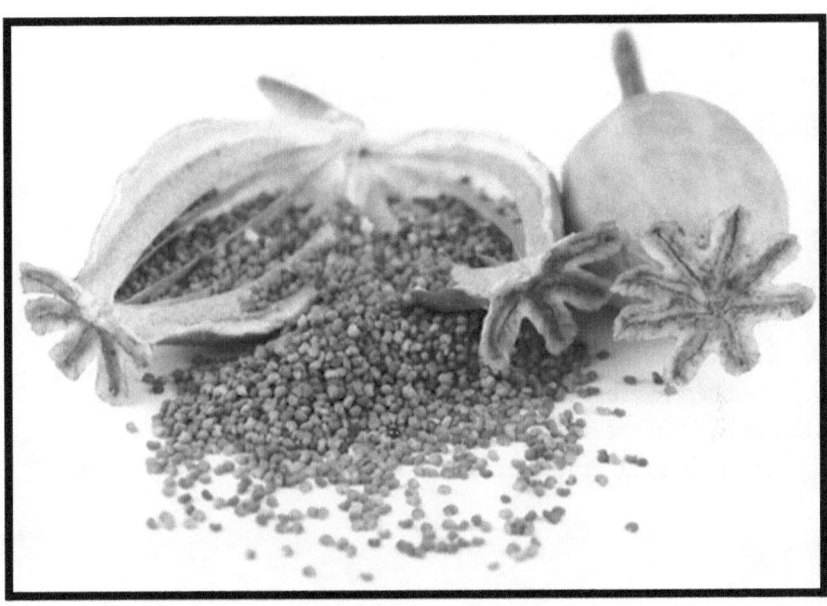

Poppy seeds are obtained from the poppy heads of the poppy plant that yields opium from the fluid inside the unripe capsules. The poppy plant originated in East Mediterranean region and Asia Minor. It was referred to by Sumerians as 'the joy plant' 3,000 years ago. Today, it is produced in both East and West countries.

Poppy plant is produced mainly for its narcotic effect. Poppy seeds contain a small quantity of morphine and codeine, enough to show up as a false positive result in athletic contests. Consuming large quantities of poppy seeds could cause hallucination.

Poppy seeds come in several colours (white, grey, blue, and black) and are tiny kidney-shaped oily seeds with a nutty flavour and aroma. Poppy seeds contain protein, oleic acid, linoleic acid (Omega-6 fatty acid), vitamins E and B, calcium, copper, iron, manganese, magnesium, zinc, selenium, potassium, and fibre.

The seeds are used whole or ground, as a spice, a condiment, a thickener, and a main ingredient in baked goods, desserts, and dishes, or pressed to yield oil.

Some of the benefits of poppy seeds are that they

1. relieve symptoms of cough and asthma.
2. aid in cardiovascular health.
3. lower the risk of breast cancer.
4. fight insomnia.
5. relieve joint swelling and pain.
6. treat diarrhoea.
7. boost energy.
8. aid in digestion.
9. are used to treat boils and nose bleed in Iran.
10. are used in tooth cavities to relieve pain in Algeria.
11. are used as an aphrodisiac.

PUMPKIN SEEDS

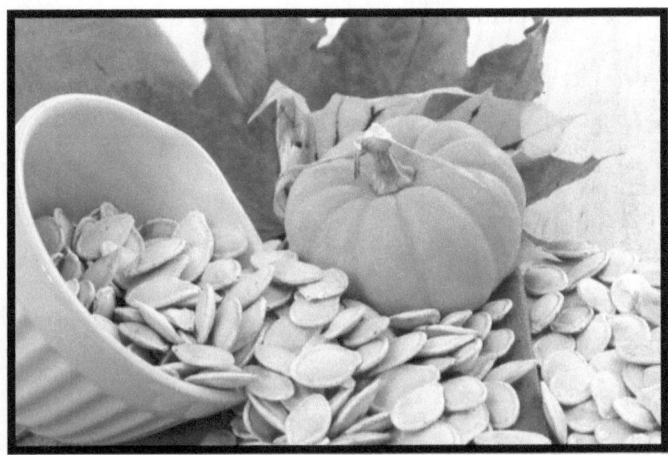

Pumpkin seed is native to the Americas, but today, China is the largest producer. It has been discovered in Mexican caves dating back to 7000 BC.

Pumpkin seed is flat and dark green with a yellowish white shell. It has a sweet nutty flavour. Pumpkin seed is high in calories (559 calories/100 g), protein, tryptophan, vitamins (E and B), minerals (manganese, magnesium, phosphorus, copper, zinc, iron, and selenium), polyphenols, phytosterols, lignans, essential fatty acids, and fibre.

Some of the benefits of pumpkin seeds are that they

1. have anticancer properties, especially against prostate and breast cancers.
2. have anti-inflammatory properties that lower pain from arthritis.
3. have antioxidant properties due to the presence of phytosterols, lignans, essential fatty acids, vitamin E, manganese, and zinc.
4. have antimicrobial properties.
5. protect prostate due to the presence of zinc, lignans, and phytosterols.
6. help maintain skin health due to the presence of zinc, selenium, essential fatty acids, and vitamin E.
7. have antidepressant and sleeping properties due to the presence of tryptophan.

8. protect heart due to the presence of unsaturated fatty acids and fibre.

9. protect bones due to the presence of minerals.

10. have alkalinity. Pumpkin seeds are the only seeds that are alkaline-forming. Most snacks are acid-forming in the body. Acidity is linked with pain and heartburn.

QUINOA SEEDS

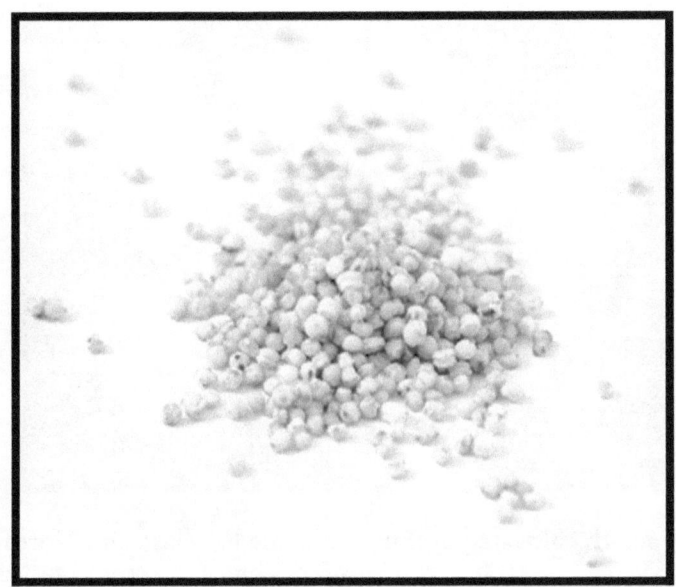

Although quinoa (pronounced keen-wa) is referred to as a grain, it is actually a seed from a vegetable related to Swiss chard, spinach, and beets.

Quinoa originated in South America 5,000 years ago.

The seeds are processed to remove the bitter coating containing saponins. Quinoa is cooked like rice and can be added to many dishes. It has a nutty taste and chewy texture.

It is high in complete protein (19 per cent) containing all the essential amino acids, including lysine, which is missing in grains, oleic acid, Omega-3 fatty acids, B vitamins, fibre, minerals (manganese, magnesium, iron, phosphorus, and copper), complex carbohydrates, and antioxidants (quercetin and kaempferol).

Quinoa has anti-inflammatory, antioxidant, and anticancer properties.

SAFFLOWER SEEDS

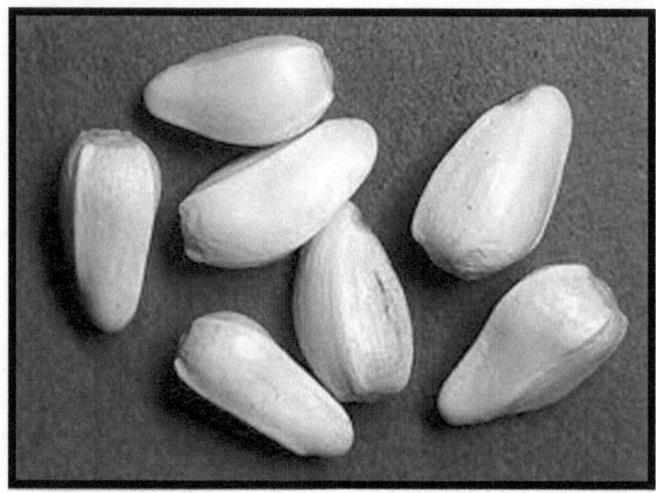

Safflower is a herb cultivated in Iran, India, the Far East, and North America.

The seeds are bitter and resemble orange seeds. The seeds and flowers are used as medicine.

The seeds are rich in oleic acid, essential fatty acids, and vitamin E. The seeds produce oil that is similar to olive oil but has a high smoking point than olive oil, making it stable in cooking at high temperatures. The oil has a light texture with a delicate flavour, is non-greasy, and can be easily absorbed.

The benefits of eating safflower seeds are that they

1. prevent heart diseases and stroke.
2. maintain healthy hair and skin.
3. have a laxative effect and prevent constipation.
4. aid in losing weight.
5. improve sex life.
6. treat cough and asthma.
7. curb premenstrual discomfort.
8. regulate blood glucose.
9. relieve pain associated with traumatic injuries.

Sesame Seeds

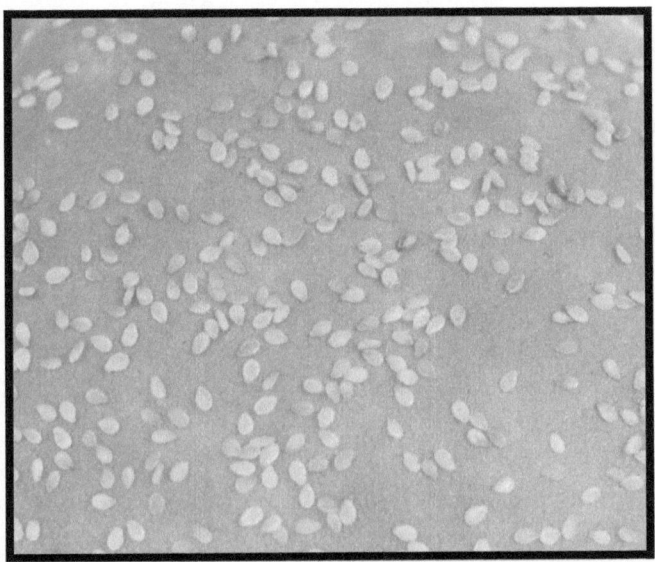

Sesame is one of the oldest cultivated plants in the world. It was cultivated for its oil more than 5,000 years ago. Nowadays, the largest producers are India, Mexico, and China. The oil is resistant to rancidity. Sesame seeds originated in India. It is the oldest condiment and had been used for food, medicine, and cosmetics. The famous magical command 'open sesame' from the tale 'Ali Baba and the Forty Thieves' in *The Arabian Nights* is familiar to all of us. It refers to the opening of seed pods at maturity.

Women in Babylon used it to prolong youth and beauty. Roman soldiers used it for stamina and strength.

Sesame seeds are tiny, flat, and oval with a nutty taste and come in several colours (white, yellow, brown, black, and red). A single pod may contain more than 100 kernels.

Sesame seeds contain lignans (sesamin and sesamolin), protein, tryptophan, fibre, oleic acid (50 per cent of its oil), vitamins (E and thiamine), minerals (calcium, magnesium, phosphorus, manganese, iron, zinc, selenium, and copper), high energy (573 calories/100 g), and phytosterols. They are the richest source of phytosterols among all the nuts and seeds. Lignans are plant estrogens that also act as antioxidants.

Sesame seeds are used in making sweet (halvah), tahini (roasted sesame seed paste), and hummus (fried sesame seed). They are sprinkled over salads, sweets, desserts, and baked products.

Some of the benefits of sesame seeds are that they

1. contain sesamine, which has estrogenic properties that inhibit the proliferation of cancer cells of leukaemia, multiple myeloma, colon, prostate, breast, pancreas, and lung.
2. Contain compounds which lower blood pressure and bad cholesterol and prevent plaque formation in the arteries.
3. promote bone health.
4. promote skin health.
5. prevent hangover by protecting the liver from alcohol damage and detoxifying the harmful substances that result from alcohol effect.
6. prevent constipation.
7. boost oral health and remove dental plaque.
8. Contain lignans, which protect the liver from oxidative damage.
9. have antidepressant effect owing to lignans and tryptophan.
10. promote asthma relief.
11. Contain magnesium, which prevents urinary spasm in asthmatics.
12. relieve postmenopausal symptoms.
13. prevent osteoporosis.
14. Can be used to massage infants to improve their sleep.

SUNFLOWER SEEDS

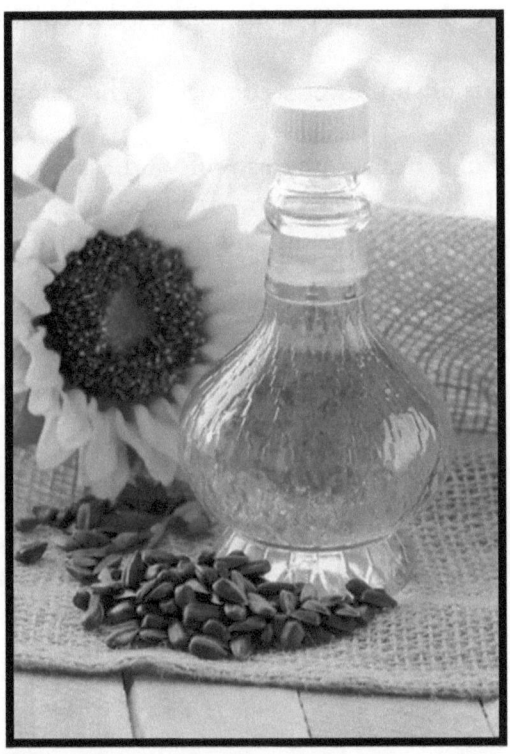

The sunflower seed originated in South America and was used by Native Americans more than 5,000 years ago. The leading producers are Russia, Peru, Argentina, Spain, and China.

Sunflower seeds come from the yellow flower that is actually 1,000-2,000 individual flowers joined together at the stem. Each flower head can produce up to 2,000 seeds.

The name sunflower comes from the fact that the flowering head turns towards the sun. The seeds are greyish white enclosed in black shells with white stripes. The seeds have a sweet nutty taste.

Sunflower seeds are rich in vitamins E and B, fibre, essential fatty acids, protein (21 per cent), tryptophan, manganese, copper, magnesium, phosphorus, selenium, and polyphenolic antioxidants.

Sunflower oil is one of the most popular oils used in cooking.

Some of the benefits of sunflower seeds include the following:

1. Cardiovascular health: phytosterols and essential fatty acids lower cholesterol, and magnesium lowers blood pressure.
2. Bone health: the minerals aid in strengthening the bone and preventing osteoporosis.
3. Anti-inflammatory properties: vitamin E lowers the severity of asthma and arthritis.
4. Nerve health: tryptophan and magnesium aid in relieving stress, anxiety, and depression.
5. Skin protection: vitamin E is an antioxidant that protects the skin from the damaging effect of UV rays and free radicals.
6. Energy: sunflower seed is rich in energy (584 calories/100 g) and should be eaten in moderation to avoid weight gain.

WATERMELON SEEDS

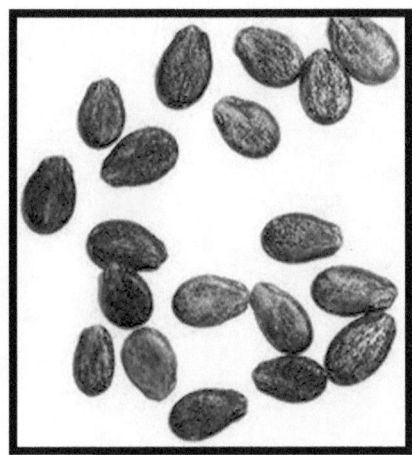

Watermelon originated in India and South Africa. It is mentioned in the Bible, and its seeds have been recovered from the tomb of Pharaoh Tutankhamun.

The seeds are red or black. They contain protein (31 g per cup), oils (50 per cent oil, mostly unsaturated), high energy (600 calories per cup), vitamin B, magnesium, phosphorus, iron, potassium, copper, manganese, and zinc.

Roasted seeds can be eaten as snack or used in soups and tea. The extract serves as a home remedy for urinary tract and stomach disorders.

The oil is used as a skin moisturiser and is an essential ingredient in body oils.

Watermelon seeds lower blood pressure and risk of coronary artery diseases.

Protein is essential for body growth and repair.

Minerals are needed for strengthening the bones.

B vitamins are necessary for good metabolism, healthy blood, and effective immune response.

So, do not spit out the seeds. Roast them and eat them to reap the benefits.

TOP FIVE HEALTHIEST SEEDS

Black Seed 'habbatul barakah'   Sesame Seed
Hemp Seed   Sunflower Seed
Pumpkin Seed

Grains (Cereals)

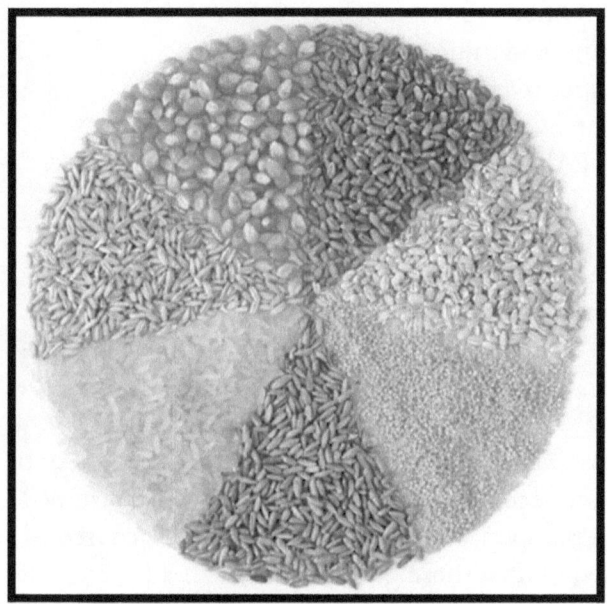

Grains are edible seeds from the grasses and come in many different sizes and shapes.

Grains are a healthy necessity in our diet. While we all know that fruits and vegetables are rich in phytonutrients and antioxidants, some of us might not be aware that whole grains are often better sources of these nutrients.

It is recommended to eat 3 oz of grains each day, at least half of which should come from whole grains.

A 1 oz serving of grain is equivalent to

    1 slice bread
    1 oz (cup) ready-to-eat cereal half a bagel muffin or bun half a cup
        cooked cereal, rice or pasta

1 pancake or wafer
6 crackers
3 cups of popcorn

Grain consists of three major parts:

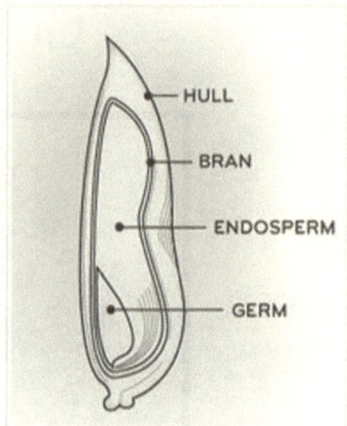

1. Bran is the outer protective layer and contains fibre, Omega-3 fatty acids, vitamins, and minerals.
2. Endosperm makes up the bulk of the grain and consists mainly of starch.
3. Germ is the smallest part of the grain from which a new plant sprouts and contains most of the nutrients such as vitamin E, folic acid, magnesium, and phosphorus.

Types of Grains

1. Whole grains: these are unrefined grains as their bran and germ have not been removed by milling: they are consumed in the form of brown rice, popcorn, brown bread, oatmeal, couscous, and bulgur.
2. Refined grains: these grains are milled, a process that removes the bran and germ to give them a finer texture and extend their shelf life; they are consumed in the form of white rice, white bread, cakes, desserts, pasta, muffins, biscuits, pancakes, waffles, and pizza.
3. Enriched grains: to these grains, some of the nutrients that are lost during processing, like folic acid, are added back.
4. Fortified grains: To these grains, some nutrients that do not occur naturally, like vitamin D, are added to augment their nutritional benefits.

Benefits of Whole Grains

1. They are low in saturated fat but high in polyunsaturated fatty acids, including Omega-3 fatty acids.
2. They are an excellent source of complex carbohydrates (starch).
3. They are high in both soluble and insoluble fibres.
4. They are a significant source of protein.

5. They are a good source of B vitamins, including folic acid.
6. They are a good source of minerals like magnesium, iron, copper, phosphorus, and zinc.
7. They are a good source of phytochemicals:

    a. Lignans can decrease the risk of heart diseases and certain cancers.
    b. Phytic acid lowers glucose absorbed from the food and decreases the risk of colon cancer.
    c. Saponins and phytosterols decrease cholesterol.
    d. Phenolic compounds have antioxidant properties.

ALPHABETICAL LIST OF GRAINS

Barley

Buckwheat

Corn

Millet

Oats

Rice

Rye

Sorghum

Spelt

Teff

Triticale

Wheat

BARLEY

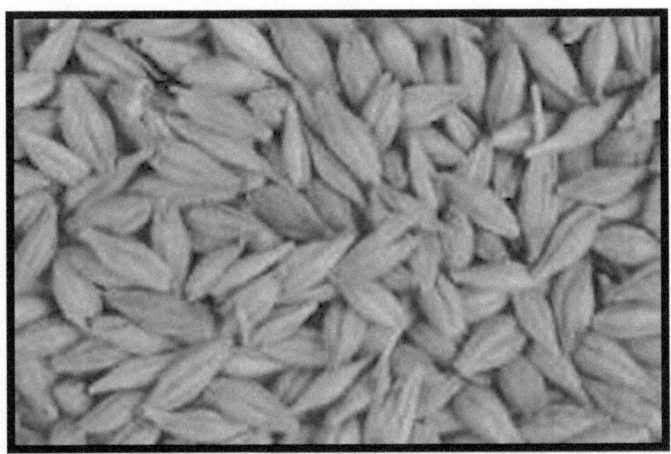

Barley originated in Ethiopia and Southeast Asia more than 10,000 years ago. The largest producers today are Canada, the United States, Russia, Germany, France, and Spain

Egyptians buried mummies with necklaces of barley.

Barley is a staple food in most countries of the Middle East, where it is used in soups and stews. In Western countries, it is mainly grown for animal feed and in the beer industry. Barley has a chewy texture, nutty flavour, and lighter colour than wheat. It is rich in fibre, niacin, selenium, copper, manganese, phosphorus, protein, tryptophan, and lignans.

Barley has many health benefits; some of them are that it

1. has fibre that lowers bad cholesterol and blood pressure.
2. has niacin that lowers the risk of heart diseases because it prevents oxidation of cholesterol by free radicals and decreases assembling of platelets, which could lead to blood clots.
3. contains fibre that also slows digestion, gives satiety, helps in weight control, and prevents constipation.
4. contains lignans that protect against breast cancer.
5. lowers the risk of diabetes type 2.

6. can help prevent gallstones.
7. protects against childhood asthma.
8. has diuretic properties, which make it beneficial in urinary and kidney conditions.
9. has tryptophan that is beneficial for insomnia, anxiety, depression, and premenstrual syndrome.
10. increases strength and endurance.
11. is beneficial in digestive disorders like diarrhoea, stomach pain, and inflammatory bowel diseases.

Buckwheat (Kasha)

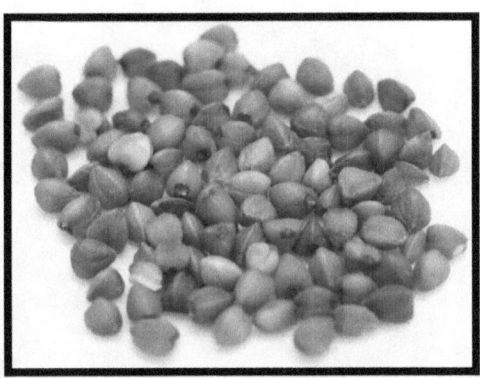

Buckwheat is not a cereal grain but a fruit seed related to rhubarb and sorrel. It is not related to wheat as it is not a grass. It is used like a grain in cooking. Its name is derived from the Dutch 'boekweit', meaning 'beech wheat', because it looks like beechnut and has the characteristics of wheat.

Buckwheat has a pink to brown colour, triangular shape, and a soft, subtle flavour. It is often served as an alternative to rice or is ground into flour.

Buckwheat originated in Northern Europe and Southeast Asia around 6000 BC, but today, it is largely produced in Russia, China, Poland, North America, and France.

Buckwheat is rich in starch, protein, fibre, phytonutrients, manganese, magnesium, and copper. Buckwheat has more protein than cereals and contains amino acids lysine and arginine, which are lacking in cereals.

Some of the health benefits of buckwheat are that it

1. lowers blood pressure and protects the heart.
2. has a low glycaemic index and lowers the risk of diabetes, unlike other cereals.
3. lowers the risk of gallstones.
4. lowers the risk of colon and breast cancers.
5. is safe for people allergic to gluten because it is gluten-free.

Corn (Maize)

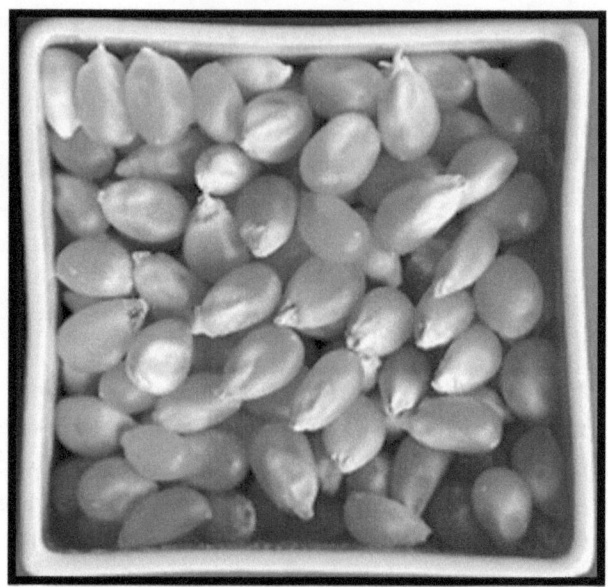

Corn is the third most important crop in the world. While corn is normally considered a vegetable, it is actually a grain. Corn originated in Central America and Mexico more than 7,000 years ago.

Unlike other cereals, corn is consumed mostly unmilled, which helps to retain all the nutrients and fibre. Corn is a staple food as tortillas, burritos, and polenta for some people and snack as popcorn, corn chip, and corn muffins for others.

Corn comes in many different colours such as white, yellow, pink, red, blue, purple, and black.

Corn is made up of 8 per cent protein, 10 per cent fat (mostly unsaturated), and 82 per cent starch. It is a good source of vitamins (B, C, and A), minerals (magnesium, manganese, iron, copper, and zinc), carotenoids (beta-carotene, lutein, and zeaxanthin), and fibre.

The high carbohydrate content is the reason for making corn syrup.

Because of its elevated fat content, it is superior to other grains as a source of energy.

Because of its high carotenoid content, vitamin C, and manganese, corn is a great antioxidant.

Its high fibre content provides numerous digestive benefits like regular bowel movement, easy digestion, prevention of haemorrhoids, and prevention of colon cancer.

Its high fibre content also regulates blood cholesterol and glucose levels.

It may be beneficial in the treatment of bed-wetting in children.

It may be beneficial for disorders of the urinary tract and prostate inflammation.

It can be used in the production of starch, glucose, and cosmetic products.

Corn oil is rich in polyunsaturated fats, which help lower blood pressure and reduce heart diseases.

Millet

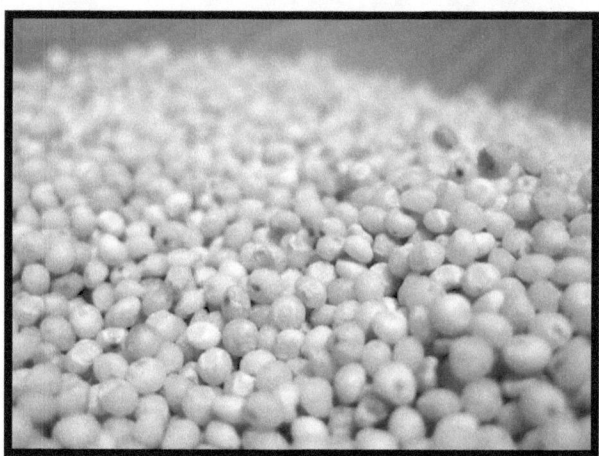

Millet is a tiny round grain with a mildly sweet and nutty flavour that comes in several colours (white, grey, yellow, and red) and many varieties (pearl, foxtail, finger, and proso or common millet).

Millet was the main grain in China before rice. Today, the majority of the world's commercial crop is produced by India, China, and Nigeria. In America and Europe, it has been grown mainly as birdseed and animal feed.

Millet ranks as the sixth most important grain in the world, sustaining one-third of the world's population. It is a significant part of the diet in China, India, and Egypt.

Millet has a hard indigestible hull that must be removed before consumption. Millet is used in flatbreads, couscous, beer, fermented drinks, and porridges. Millet is even mentioned as a treasured crop in the Bible.

It is rich in protein (15 per cent), fibre, some B vitamins, tryptophan, manganese, magnesium, phosphorus, and phytochemicals.

Millet is gluten-free and non-allergenic.

It is highly alkaline, making it easily digestible and soothing to the stomach.

It has high antioxidant activity that lowers blood cholesterol and the risk of certain cancers.

Its high magnesium content maintains normal muscle and nerve function.

It has tryptophan, which makes serotonin that calms and soothes the mood.

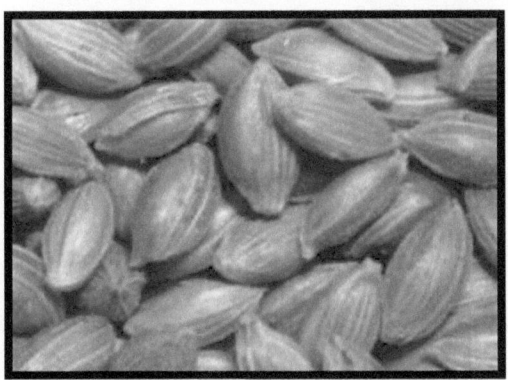

Fonio

Fonio is a tiny variety of millet, commonly eaten by inhabitants of West Africa. It comes in two varieties of white and black.

Fonio is the oldest African cereal, where it has been the staple food for thousands of years. It is one of the world's best tasting cereals.

Fonio is the most nutritious of all grains. It is richer in calcium, magnesium, zinc, and manganese than other grains. It is rich in sulphur-containing amino acids, methionine and cysteine.

Fonio is regarded as a grain with medicinal and healing properties. It is recommended for lactating women and diabetics because of its insulin-secreting properties.

OATS

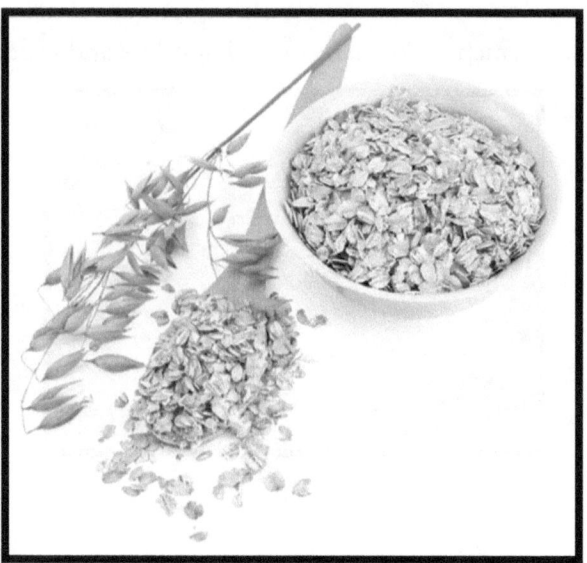

Oat originated in the Near East and cultivated in Europe, where it is an important crop. Today, the largest producers of oats include Russia, the United States, Germany, Poland, and Finland. Oats can be rolled, flaked, or made into oat meal or flour for porridge and bread. Oatmeal is a finely milled oat grain that contains vitamin E and fat.

Oats contain vitamin B, manganese, phosphorus, magnesium, iron, zinc, selenium, starch, fibre, protein, lignans, and beta-glucan. It is the only cereal containing a globulin protein (avenalin) as the major storage protein. Oat protein is considered as good as soy and animal proteins. The protein content of oat is up to 24 per cent, which is the highest among all cereals.

Eating oats is considered a healthy habit because of the many health benefits it has; some of them are that it

1. lowers bad cholesterol, blood pressure, and heart diseases.
2. contains more soluble fibre than any other grain, resulting in slower digestion and an extended sensation of fullness; thus, it is good for weight control.

3. increases the hormones that control appetite.
4. has beta-glucan, which boosts immunity.
5. contains lignans, which protect against breast cancer and heart diseases.
6. stabilises blood glucose and lowers the risk of diabetes type 2.
7. improves athletic performance by its carbohydrates which provide energy.
8. lowers the risk of gall bladder stones.
9. lowers the risk of colon and stomach cancers.
10. prevents constipation.
11. can help with sleep.

RICE

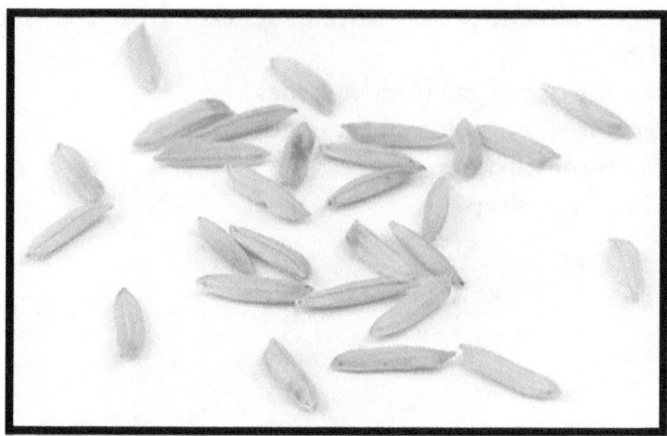

Rice originated in China more than 4,000 years ago. Today, rice is the most consumed staple food in Asia and West Indies. One-half of the world's population depend on it as their staple food. It provides 20 per cent of the world's dietary energy supply as compared to 19 per cent for wheat and 5 per cent for corn.

Types of Rice

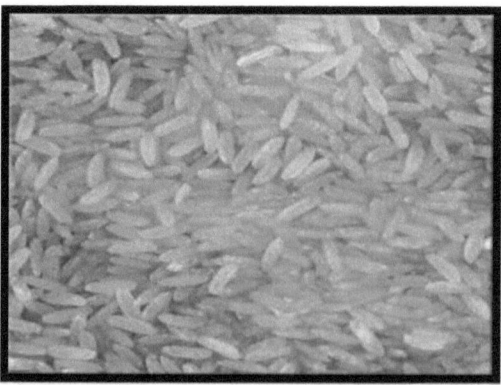

Brown rice: only the husk is removed, but the bran and germ are retained. It is high in fibre, protein, vitamin B, iron, manganese, magnesium, and a small quantity of fat.

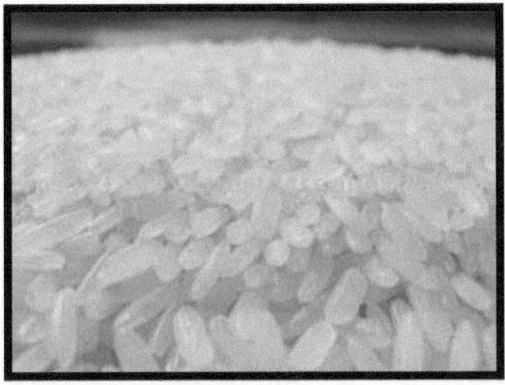

White rice: it is obtained after milling and polishing to remove husk, bran, and germ. This process alters the flavour, appearance, texture, and nutritional content of the grain, leaving only the starch of endosperm. White rice must be enriched with iron, thiamine, and niacin during processing; otherwise, it would lead to deficiency symptoms.

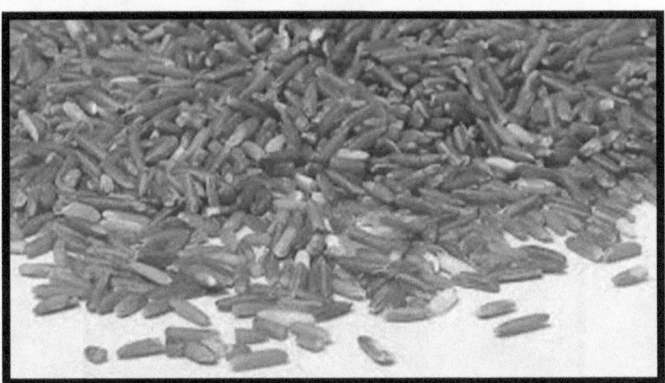

Red rice: it is unhulled or partially hulled rice with intact germ and has a red husk. It is grown for its red colour, nutty taste, and high nutritional value. When red rice is cooked, the natural red colour in the bran or hull leaches out and dyes the rest of the dish pink or red. Red rice is grown in Southeast Asia, Europe, and the Southern United States.

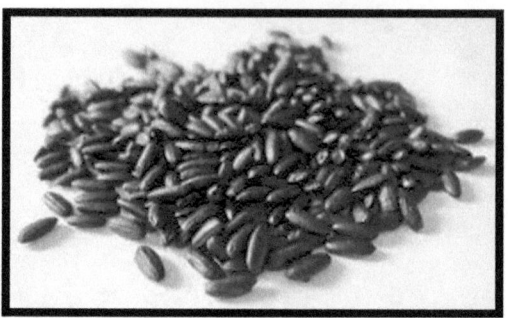

Black rice: it is an unmilled medium grain with black bran which turns deep purple when cooked. In West Bengal, India, there is another variety of black rice that turns white on cooking. Black rice has a mild nutty taste. It is used in porridge and desserts. It is rich in the health-promoting antioxidant anthocyanin, similar to that found in blueberries and blackberries.

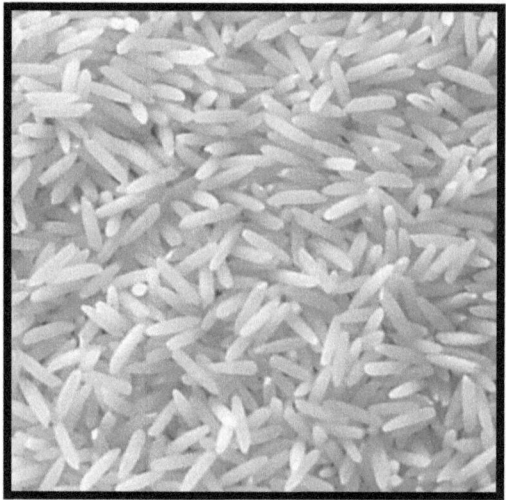

Basmati rice: it is considered the 'prince of rice' and is grown in the Himalayas and Pakistan. It has a long grain with a light nutty flavour and pleasant fragrance. After cooking, it becomes longer, lighter, and more fluffy, and the grains do not stick together. Basmati rice is a good choice for curries, biryani, and pulao.

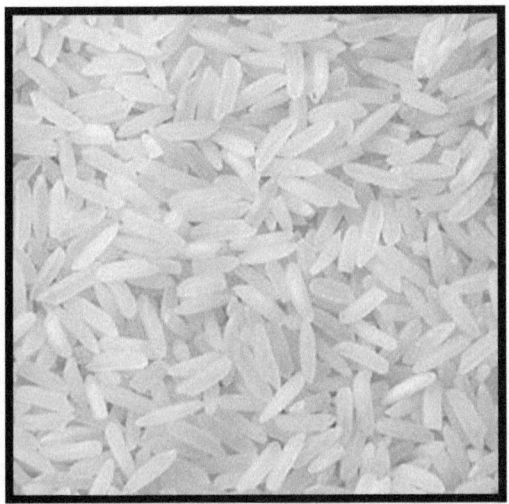

Jasmine rice: it is known as 'Thai fragrant rice'. It is a fragrant variety of a long grain rice grown in Thailand. It has a light fluffy texture and nutty flavour. After cooking, it gives a delicate jasmine scent.

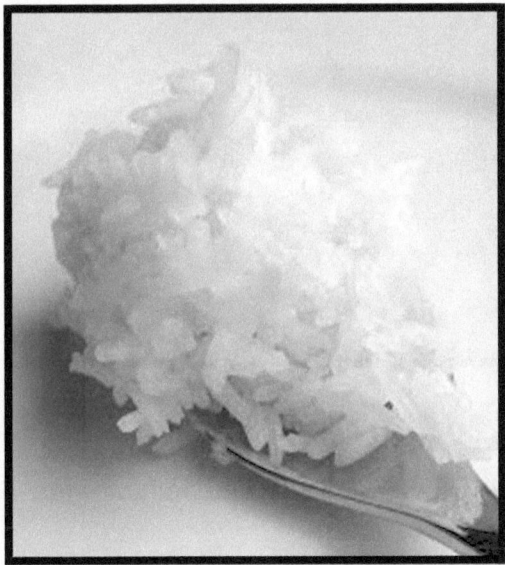

Sticky rice: it is also known as glutinous or sweet rice. It is opaque round rice that has a starchy glue-like waxy texture. This is due to the absence of the amylose portion of the starch. Other types of rice have both amylose and amylopectin. Sticky rice is used to make sweets and rice dumplings. It is grown mainly in Southeast and East Asia.

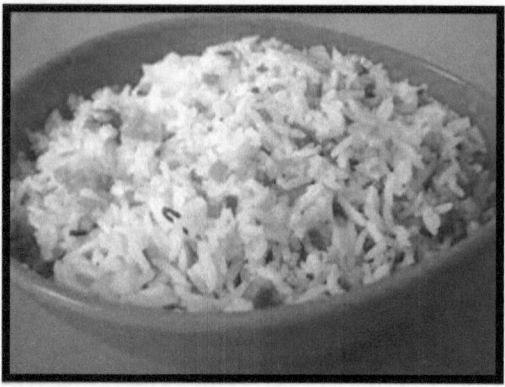

Fried rice: it is made from steamed rice that is stir-fried in a wok, often together with other ingredients like egg, vegetables, prawn, chicken, and meat.

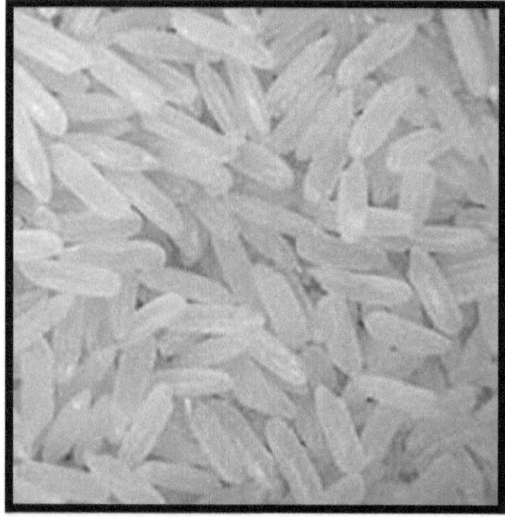

Parboiled rice: this rice is steeped in hot water overnight prior to the removal of hull and bran. This process allows nutrients to push inside the grain, making it more nutritious than the common white rice.

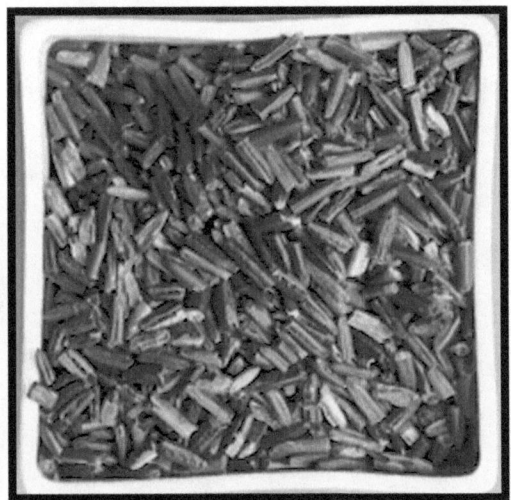

Wild rice: it is also known as Indian rice because it was a popular food of the American Indians. It is the only grain native to North America. Wild rice is not a true grain but the seed of an aquatic grass. The seeds have a nutty flavour and chewy texture. They are much larger, denser, and more nutritious than the common rice.

Brown rice has the following additional advantages as compared to white rice:

1. It lowers cholesterol and protects the heart.
2. It lowers the risk of diabetes type 2.
3. It lowers the risk of colon cancer.
4. It helps prevent gallstones.
5. It protects against childhood asthma.

Rye

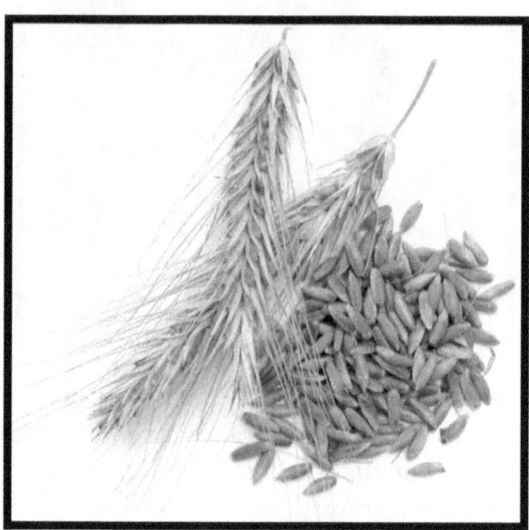

Rye is a grain closely related to barley and wheat but is longer and more slender. It has a deep hardy taste and varies in colour from greyish green to yellowish brown.

Rye grows wild in Turkey. It was first cultivated in Germany. Today, the major cultivators are Russia, China, Denmark, Canada, and Poland.

Rye is a rich source of protein, fibre, some B vitamins, manganese, phosphorus, magnesium, lignans, and fructans (fructose polymer) as its main sugar source. It has lower gluten content than wheat.

Rye is used for flour, bread, alcoholic beverages, and animal fodder. Rye flour has more nutrients than refined wheat because it is difficult to separate bran and germ from the rye kernel.

Some of the benefits of rye are that it

1. lowers bad cholesterol and blood pressure, thus protects the heart.
2. improves insulin sensitivity, controls blood sugar, and lowers the risk of type 2 diabetes.

3. protects against certain cancers, such as colon, prostate, and breast cancers.
4. supports gastrointestinal health and prevents constipation.
5. may ease postmenopausal symptoms like hot flashes.
6. assists in weight control.
7. helps in the prevention of gallstones.
8. protects against childhood asthma.

SORGHUM

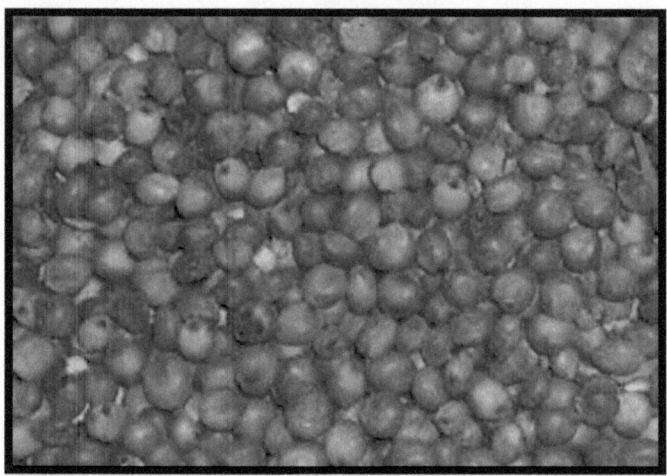

Sorghum is an important grain used for porridge, couscous, syrup, molasses, forage, beer, and ethanol as car fuel.

Sorghum originated in Egypt around 8000 BC. Now, the United States is the largest producer of sorghum. Sorghum is the fifth most produced grain in the world besides wheat, corn, rice, and barley.

Sorghum has a slightly sweet taste and comes in several colours (white, red, and black). It is usually eaten with the hull (outer layer of the grain) which retains the majority of nutrients.

Sorghum is rich in fibre, protein, B vitamins, potassium, magnesium, manganese, and more antioxidants than oat and wheat. Sorghum bran has greater antioxidant and anti-inflammatory properties than famous fruits such as blueberries and pomegranate.

Sorghum is gluten-free and is a great substitute for those allergic to gluten.

Sorghum lowers the risk of heart diseases, diabetes type 2, and certain cancers (colon and skin).

Spelt

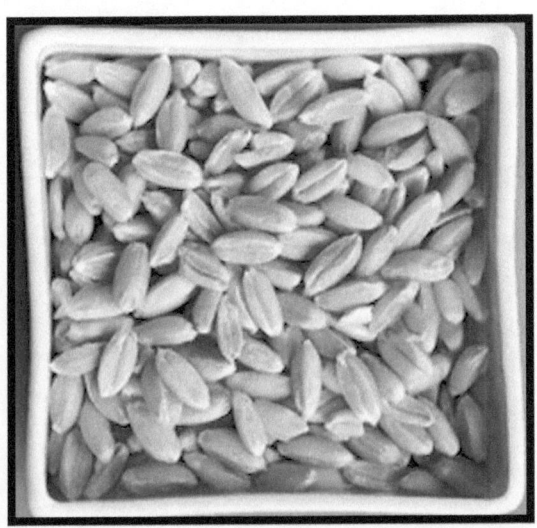

Spelt is an ancient grain which is a distant relative to the common wheat but has more protein and B vitamins than wheat. It can be used as wheat in making pasta and bread.

Spelt was cultivated by ancient civilisations in the Middle East and Southeast Europe more than 7,000 years ago. Spelt is even mentioned in the Bible.

Spelt is covered by a tough outer husk which requires removal in a further process before the grain can be milled into flour, thus making it more expensive than wheat.

Spelt has a nutty flavour and can make fantastic bread and delicious pastries.

It is a good source of fibre, protein, B vitamins, manganese, phosphorus, magnesium, copper, and zinc.

Spelt is gluten-free, so it can be used as a substitute for people sensitive to wheat gluten.

It lowers the risk of heart diseases.

It lowers the risk of type 2 diabetes.

It protects against breast cancer.

It protects against childhood asthma.

It prevents gallstones.

It lowers the occurrence of migraine headaches.

TEFF (LOVEGRASS)

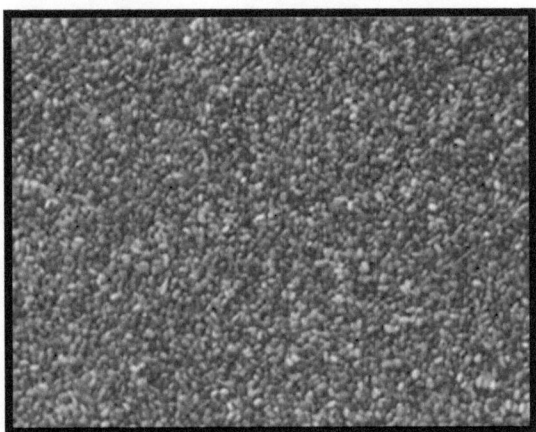

Teff is a tiny grain (less than 1 mm in diameter), similar to poppy seeds. The word teff means 'lost' due to its tiny size. Teff grains are the smallest grains in the world. A single grain of wheat weighs as much as 150 teff grains.

Teff originated in Ethiopia around 4000 BC. Today, it accounts for one-fourth of the total cereal production in Ethiopia.

Teff grain is sweet and nutty and varies in colour from white to brown to red. Although people prefer the white variety, it is the red which has the highest quantity of iron.

Because teff grain is so tiny, it is impossible to remove bran and germ from the kernel during processing. Hence, teff is a very nutritious grain because it retains all its fibre and nutrients.

Teff is eaten as sour-dough bread, waffles, pancakes, snacks, soups, and stews.

Teff is rich in protein (14 per cent), fibre, calcium, phosphorus, iron, copper, manganese, magnesium, zinc, and vitamin B1. Its protein content is higher than wheat and barley and is gluten-free, making it a great substitute for those allergic to gluten. Teff protein consists largely of easily digestible albumins (similar to egg white protein).

Teff is also free of phytic acid, which inhibits absorption of nutrients from the gut.

It has high iron content, especially in the red variety, which prevents anaemia.

It controls blood glucose level.

It has energy-enhancing properties and is favoured by athletes.

TRITICALE

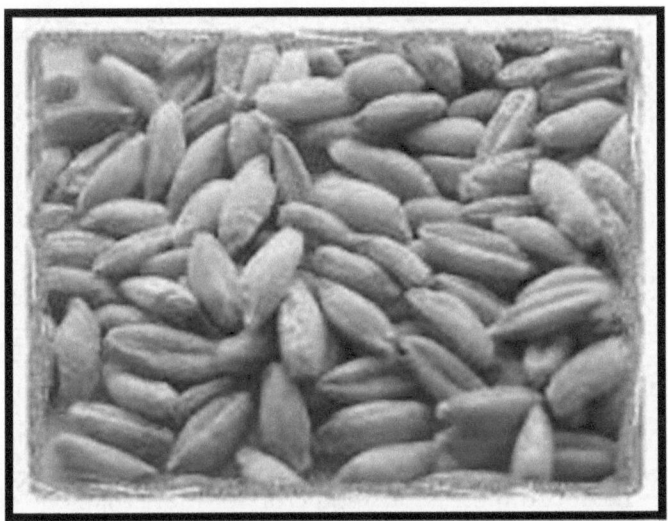

This grain is a hybrid between wheat and rye. It was first produced in the nineteenth century in Scotland and Sweden. Plant breeders hoped to get a new crop with higher yield and better resistance. However, the product is inferior in quality to wheat although it is superior to rye.

Triticale is mostly used as animal feed.

WHEAT

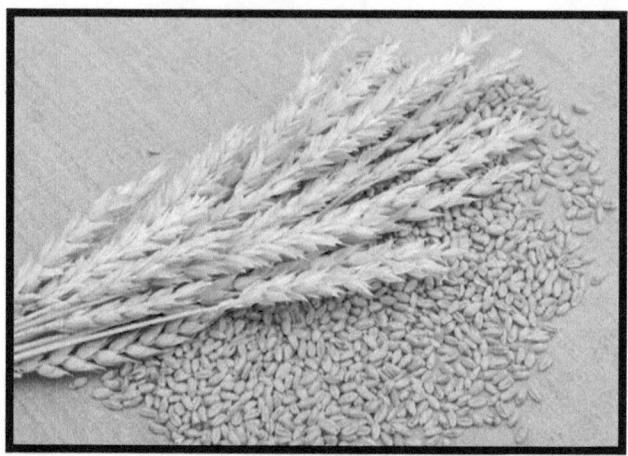

Wheat is the most common staple food crop for more than one-third of the world's population. Wheat originated from Southwest Asia around 8000 BC. Now, it is grown all over the world.

Wheat grain is oval and rounded at both ends. Wheat kernels can be red or white. The red variety has more strong-flavoured tannins than the milder white variety.

It is a good source of protein (gluten), fibre, B vitamins, vitamin E, starch, lutein, zeaxanthin, phytosterols, and minerals (zinc, iron, magnesium, phosphorus, and selenium).

Hard wheat is rich in protein and is used principally in breads and pastas. Soft wheat has lower protein content and is used mainly to make cakes, biscuits, and pastry.

Some of the benefits of eating bread include the following:

1. It provides slow release of glucose and is thus helpful in preventing type 2 diabetes.
2. It provides energy. Seventy per cent of the calorie intake of the world's population is from wheat.

3. Its low fat and high fibre content lower the risk of heart diseases. Vitamin E prevents the oxidation of bad cholesterol, thus preventing the blockage of arteries.
4. Its fibre protects against colon cancer, and its phytosterols lower the risk of breast cancer.
5. It has the carotenoids lutein and zeaxanthin, which protect the eye and skin.
6. Wheat germ oil helps in the case of irregular menopausal symptoms.

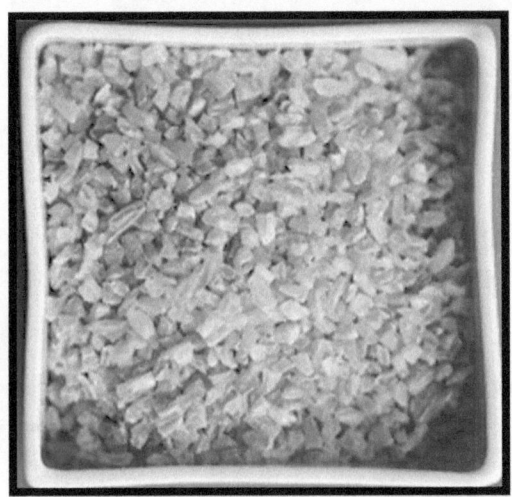

Bulgur

Bulgur, a Turkish word, results from parboiling, drying, and crushing the wheat kernel. Only a very small amount of bran is removed. It cooks very quickly.

It has a light nutty flavour and can be used in pilaffs, soups, bakery products, or stuffings. Bulgur is the main ingredient in Middle Eastern dishes, such as tabbouleh, kibbeh, and jarish.

Bulgur is high in fibre and protein but low in fat and calories. It offers numerous health benefits and is ideal for including in weight management diets.

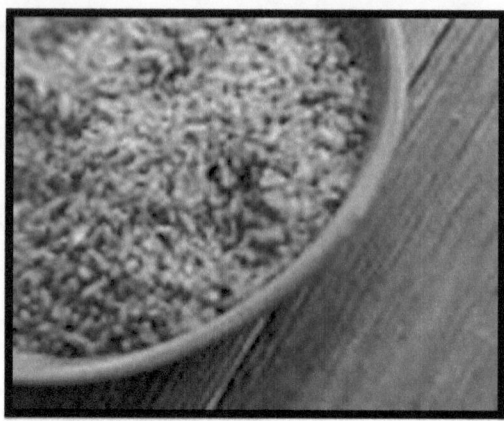

Freekeh (Farik)

Freekeh is whole wheat that has been harvested while still green and young, then roasted and cracked. It is used in a number of dishes across the Middle East.

Freekeh is very nutritious with high protein and fibre content.

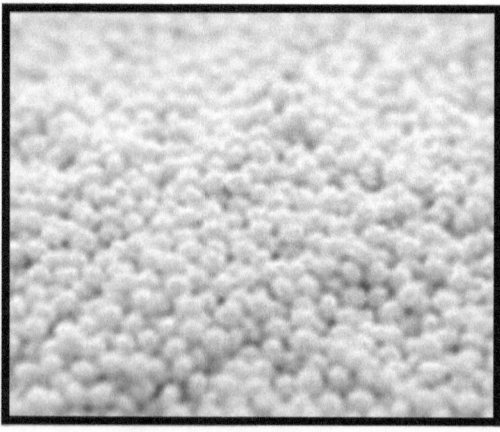

Couscous

Couscous consists of many tiny granules made from steamed and dried whole wheat. It has a nutty flavour and chewy texture. Couscous is a popular alternative to rice and pasta in North African countries and is a staple of Morocco.

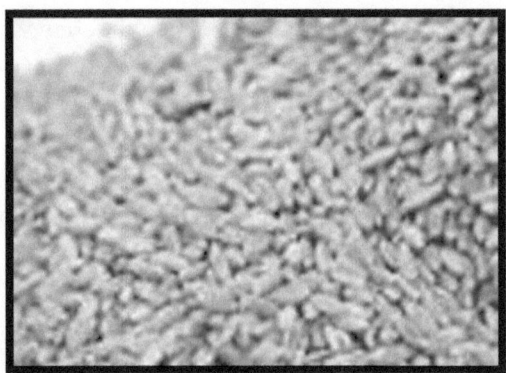

Wheatberries

Wheatberries are whole unprocessed wheat kernels that contain all the three parts of the grain, including bran, endosperm, and germ. Only the inedible outer hull has been removed. Thus, they retain all the grain's phytonutrients, fibre, vitamins, and minerals.

Wheatberries look like thick, short grain with a nutty flavour and chewy texture.

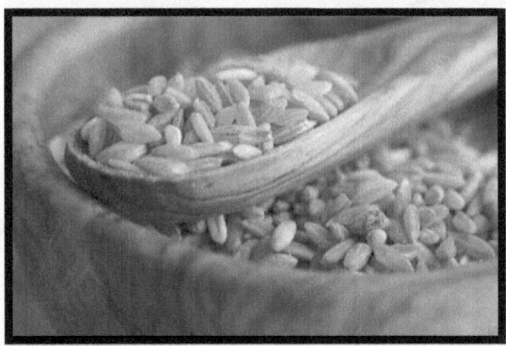

Farro

Farro is the Near Eastern mother grain from which all other grains were derived thousands of years ago.

It looks like spelt, but unlike spelt that can be boiled straight off, farro must be soaked first. After cooking, farro will give a firm chewy texture, whereas spelt softens and becomes mushy.

Farro is a nutty, slightly sweet, and pleasingly chewy grain. It is tastier than spelt or kamut. It is a popular grain in Italy, parts of Europe, Asia, and the Middle East.

It is a whole grain that has twice the fibre and protein of modern wheat. The gluten content of farro is weaker than modern wheat, making it more digestible.

Farro is an excellent source of a specific carbohydrate called cyanogenic glycosides that stimulate the immune system, lower cholesterol, and control blood sugar.

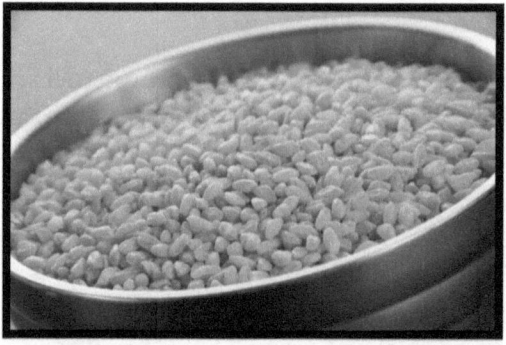

Grano

Grano, which means grain in Italian, originated in Southern Italy. It results from lightly polishing wheat; hence, it retains most of its fibre, protein, and other nutrients. It has a golden hue and dense texture and tastes like pasta.

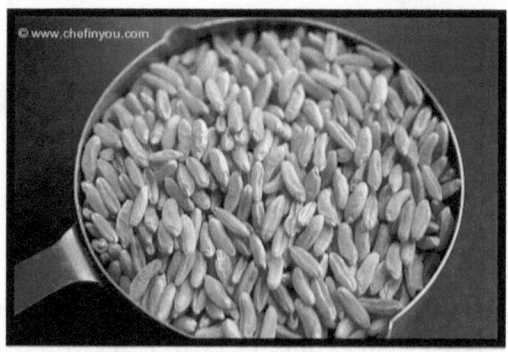

Kamut (Khorasan Wheat)

Kamut, which means wheat in the ancient Egyptian language, is a whole grain related to wheat but two to three times the size of the wheat grain. It has more protein, fibre, fatty acids, vitamins, and minerals than common wheat. Kamut has a sweet nutty flavour and chewy texture. It can be incorporated in pasta, cereals, and salads.

TOP FIVE HEALTHIEST GRAINS

Barley   Oat
Buckwheat   Rye
Millet

TOP FIVE MOST PRODUCED GRAINS

Wheat	Barley
Corn	Sorghum
Rice	

www.ingramcontent.com/pod-product-compliance
Lightning Source LLC
Chambersburg PA
CBHW022001170526
45157CB00003B/1098